Living with
Diabetes

Living with Diabetes

The Diabetes UK Guide for those Treated with Diet and Tablets

New Edition

Dr John L. Day
The Ipswich Hospital, UK

JOHN WILEY & SONS, LTD

Chichester • New York • Weinheim • Brisbane • Singapore • Toronto

First published 1998 by John Wiley & Sons Ltd, Baffins Lane, Chichester, West Sussex
PO19 1UD, England
New Edition published 2001
  National   01243 779777   International   (+44) 1243 779777
  e-mail (for orders and customer service enquiries): cs-books@wiley.co.uk
  Visit our Home Page on http://www.wiley.co.uk or http://www.wiley.com

Other Wiley Editorial Offices

John Wiley & Sons, Inc., 605 Third Avenue, New York, NY 10158-0012, USA

WILEY-VCH Verlag GmbH, Pappelallee 3, D-69469 Weinheim, Germany

John Wiley & Sons Australia Ltd, 33 Park Road, Milton, Queensland 4064, Australia

John Wiley & Sons (Asia) Pte Ltd, 2 Clementi Loop #02-01, Jin Xing Distripark, Singapore 129809

John Wiley & Sons (Canada) Ltd, 22 Worcester Road, Rexdale, Ontario M9W 1L1, Canada

Library of Congress Cataloging-in-Publication Data

Day, John L. (John Leigh)
    Living with diabetes : the Diabetes UK guide for those treated with diet and tablets /
John L. Day
    p. cm.
    Previous ed. had subtitle: British Diabetic Association guide for those treated with diet
and tablets.
    Includes index.
    ISBN 0-471-48713-9
    1. Non-insulin-dependent diabetes—Popular works. I. Diabetes UK. II. Title.

  RC662. 18.D38 2001
  616.4'62—dc21   2001026765

British Library Cataloguing in Publication Data

A catalogue record for this book is available from the British Library

ISBN 0-471-48713-9

Typeset in 11/13 pt Plantin from the author's disks by
Hilite Design & Reprographics Ltd, Southampton, Hampshire
Graphical illustrations by Ann Postill Technical Tracing & Allied Services, Guildford, Surrey;
Medical illustrations by Peter Lamb, Lamda Science Artwork, Corfu, Greece; Cartoons by
Clinton Banbury, Illustration & Design, Billericay, Essex
Printed and bound in Great Britain by L & S Printing Company Ltd, Worthing, West Sussex
This book is printed on acid-free paper responsibly manufactured from sustainable forestry, in
which at least two trees are planted for each one used for paper production.

Contents

Acknowledgements vii

1 **Introducing Diabetes** 1
    About diabetes 1

2 **Type 2 (Non Insulin Dependent) Diabetes** 9
    So what happens when you develop diabetes? 9
    Who gets diabetes? Why? 15

3 **Food and Physical Activity** 21
    Eliminate symptoms 21
    Prevent late complications 21
    The steps you need to take 22
    What will the diet be like? 23
    Healthy eating – putting it into practice 29
    Exercise – part of your treatment 43
    Summary 45

4 **Tablet Treatment** 47
    Which tablets? 47
    Some important questions about tablet treatment 48
    Summary 50

5 **Is Your Treatment Effective?** 51
    Blood tests versus urine tests 51
    Urine tests 52
    Overall assessment of your blood glucose 52
    Blood tests 57
    Regular weighing 58
    When diabetes goes out of control 58
    Summary 60

6 **Insulin Treatment** 63
    Why injections? 64
    Insulin treatment 64
    Summary 68

7 **The Long-Term Effects of Diabetes and Your General Health 69**
    Arterial disease and high blood pressure 70
    Damage to the feet 71
    Sexual function 76
    Other rare problems due to neuropathy 77
    Damage to the eyes 77
    Damage to the kidneys 79
    Diabetes and other illnesses 79
    Clinic attendance 82
    Regular medical review 82
    Summary 85

8 **Diabetes and Your Daily Life 87**
    Employment 87
    Financial implications of having diabetes 89
    Driving 91
    Exercise and sport 93
    Retirement 94
    Travel and holidays 95
    Contraception, pregnancy and parenthood 98
    The effect on your family 99
    Who is available to help? 100
    Some final comments on diabetes and your everyday life 100

9 **Diabetes UK 103**
    Diabetes UK's history 104
    Providing care and advice 104
    Sharing experiences 107
    Spreading the word 108
    Fighting discrimination 110
    Leading the way to better care 112
    Searching for a cure 113
    How you can help 114
    How to join Diabetes UK 116
    National and regional offices 117

Index 121

Acknowledgements

I wish to acknowledge the important contributions to this book from J Rowley BSc SRD, Dietitian, and A Blain SRN, Senior Specialist Nurse, both of the Ipswich Diabetes Centre and, in particular, E Bartlett (Diabetes UK) who has been responsible for many of the amendments in this edition.

Copyright of *The Balance of Good Health Plate* on page 29 is held by the Health Education Authority, Trevelyan House, 30 Great Peter Street, London SW1 2HW, and it is reproduced here by their kind permission.

'A lot' and 'A little' figures on page 38 reproduced by permission of MAFF (now Department for Environment, Food & Rural Affairs) from Foodsense booklet *Use Your Label* (PB2362 – © Crown copyright).

The self-check height and weight chart on page 41 is reproduced by permission from J S Garrow, 1981, *Treat Obesity Seriously*, published by Churchill Livingstone, Edinburgh, with acknowledgement to The Health Education Council, E Fullard, Oxford, and Servier Laboratories Limited, UK.

The illustration of the Active Erection Assistance System on page 76 was kindly supplied by Genesis Medical (Sales) Limited, 7 Heathgate Place, Agincourt Road, London NW3 2NU, and is reproduced here by their kind permission.

1 Introducing Diabetes

■ About diabetes

The purpose of this book

Diabetes or, to give it its full name, diabetes mellitus, is very common. In the United Kingdom there are 1.4 million people known to have diabetes, of whom 20 000 are aged under 20. Diabetes UK believes that there may be as many as another 1 million people who remain undiagnosed. Worldwide there are over 151 million cases.

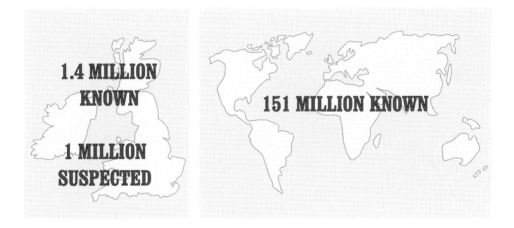

The estimated numbers of people with diabetes

Diabetes cannot be cured. However, you will see that there are steps you can take to ensure that the effects on your life are kept to a minimum.

You may wish to know more about the causes of diabetes to avoid undue worry that it is your own, or somebody else's, fault.

The aim of this book is to encourage you: to follow the recommended treatment with optimism; to share your concerns with those available to help; to be able to discuss your diabetes and its effects freely and without embarrassment with your friends, relatives and colleagues; and to attend regularly for the medical checks that are necessary from time to time.

If you are reading this book, either you have discovered that you have diabetes, or you are finding out more to help a relative or friend. You are not expected to read the book from cover to cover, but you may wish just to check on certain details or to refresh your memory on some aspects. The chapters have been divided with these possibilities in mind.

What is diabetes?

Diabetes is a disorder in which the mechanism for converting glucose to energy no longer functions properly. This causes an abnormally high level of glucose in the blood, giving rise to a variety of symptoms. If the glucose levels remain high over several years, damage may be caused to various parts of the body. Treatment of diabetes is designed not only to reverse symptoms but also to prevent any serious problems developing later.

How does diabetes develop?

Normally, the amount of glucose in the body is very carefully controlled. We obtain glucose from the food we eat, either from sweet things or from starchy foods (carbohydrates), such as bread and potatoes. Glucose can also be made by breaking down the body stores of starch in the liver. This will occur when the body needs an extra supply of glucose. This happens if you miss several meals, or have been injured, or are unwell.

The use of glucose to provide energy requires the presence of the chemical hormone, insulin. Insulin is released into the blood as the blood glucose rises after a meal. Its function is to return the glucose concentration to its original level. Less insulin is produced when the glucose level falls, for example during exercise. Insulin plays a vital role in maintaining the correct level of blood glucose.

When there is a shortage of insulin, or if the available insulin does not function correctly, then the blood glucose rises and diabetes results.

The blood glucose level of someone who does not have diabetes normally varies between 3.5 and 9.0 mmol/l.

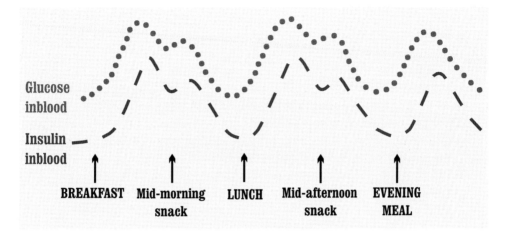

Insulin rising and falling in response to the blood glucose. This shows the blood glucose rising after each meal or snack. This rise stimulates the release of insulin. The insulin returns the glucose level to normal

A little history

Diabetes cannot be called a 'modern' condition. It was referred to in ancient Egyptian, Indian, Roman, Japanese and Chinese writings.

However, no significant advance was made in understanding the nature of diabetes until the 19th century. The first major breakthrough came in 1889. Two German scientists discovered that the removal of the pancreas, a large gland in the abdomen, gave rise to diabetes. It was also discovered that damage to clusters of cells in the pancreas, called islets of Langerhans, produced certain forms of diabetes. It was not until 1921 that two Canadians, Frederick Banting and Charles Best, made their famous discovery of insulin.

Who gets diabetes? Why?

In the United Kingdom, as many as three people in every 100 have diabetes, and perhaps one in every 600 schoolchildren. It can occur at any age, but is very rare in infants. It is more common in people approaching middle-age and in older people.

There are two main types of diabetes.

- Type 2 – Non insulin dependent diabetes.

- Type 1 – Insulin dependent diabetes.

Type 2 – Non insulin dependent diabetes

Cause

If you have Type 2 diabetes you are still producing insulin, but it is either not being made in sufficient quantities or not working properly (insulin resistance). You do not need to take insulin in order to survive. Most people with Type 2 diabetes can be treated effectively by diet, or by a combination of diet and tablets. Sometimes insulin injections may be necessary to establish good control of blood glucose levels. If you do require insulin it doesn't mean that you have developed Type 1 diabetes. It just means that you need a little more help to keep your Type 2 diabetes under control. Despite continuing research, the cause is not yet known.

Who gets it?

Type 2 diabetes used to be called 'maturity onset diabetes'. This was because it occurs mainly in the middle and older age groups, although it can sometimes occur in young people, particulary if they are not physically active. Overweight people are particularly likely to develop this type of diabetes. It tends to run in families. People from African–Caribbean and Asian backgrounds are more commonly affected. Women who have raised blood glucose levels during pregnancy are more likely to develop diasbetes in later life.

Type 1 – Insulin dependent diabetes

Cause

In this type of diabetes there is a complete or near complete absence of insulin, due to the destruction of the insulin-producing cells. With this type of diabetes it is essential to have insulin treatment to survive.

The exact cause of the damage to the insulin-producing cells is not known for certain, but a combination of factors may be involved including:

■ Damage to the insulin-producing cells by viral or other infections

■ An abnormal reaction of the body against the insulin-producing cells.

Who gets it?

In general, Type 1 diabetes is first diagnosed in younger people (under 30 years of age), but occasionally it occurs in older people, even the very old. Both sexes are equally affected.

There is some tendency for this type of diabetes to run in families, but the condition is far from being entirely inherited.

Other causes of diabetes

Diseases of the pancreas

A very few cases of diabetes are due to various diseases of the pancreas. These include inflammation (pancreatitis) or unusual deposits of iron. Mumps may sometimes have the same effect.

Accidents or illness

Major accidents or illnesses do not cause diabetes. However, they do sometimes produce a temporary increase in blood glucose.

If your diabetes was discovered during the course of an illness, it is most likely that you already had diabetes (even though you may not have had any symptoms). Some forms of hormone imbalance may also produce temporary diabetes.

Tablets

Some tablets can increase the blood glucose and reveal pre-existing diabetes. Steroid drugs or water tablets which eliminate fluid from the body (diuretics) may do this.

The contraceptive pill

This does not cause diabetes, but it may raise the blood glucose slightly.

Heredity

If one parent has Type 1 diabetes, his or her children are slightly more likely than average to develop diabetes. The risk, however, is small. For example, the chances of developing diabetes before the age of 20 are perhaps only one in 100. Rarely, both parents have diabetes, in which case the chances are increased.

Type 2 diabetes is more commonly inherited than Type 1 diabetes. However, this form usually occurs in people who are middle-aged or older, therefore their children are not usually affected until later in life. This is more likely to happen if such children become overweight when they are middle-aged.

To summarise, it is possible for someone to inherit a tendency to diabetes, but not to inherit the condition itself. This only develops because of some other influence. Thus, there are very many people with a strong family history of the disorder who never develop diabetes.

Onset of symptoms and their severity

The main symptoms of diabetes are:

- Increased thirst and a dry mouth
- Going to pass water all the time – especially at night
- Extreme tiredness
- Weight loss
- Genital itching or regular episodes of thrush
- Blurred vision.

Symptoms vary considerably in their severity and rate of onset, but they can all be rapidly relieved by treatment.

Type 2 (Non insulin dependent diabetes)

The symptoms are similar to those of Type 1 diabetes, but they develop more gradually and are usually less severe. Some people may experience no obvious symptoms. Diabetic coma does not occur in this type of diabetes.

Type 1 (Insulin dependent diabetes)

The symptoms develop fairly quickly, usually over a few weeks. Sometimes they come on quite quickly over just a few days. Without insulin treatment the condition progressively worsens, resulting in a significant weight loss, dehydration, vomiting, the onset of drowsiness and diabetic coma.

Some people with diabetes fail to notice any symptoms, but after being treated they usually have more energy and feel considerably better. Unfortunately, the presence of symptoms is no guide to the level of glucose in the blood, and it is essential that diabetes is treated, even when there are no symptoms.

Treatment

Diabetes is a very common disorder. Although no 'cure' is yet possible, all types of diabetes can be treated and normal health restored.

Treatment is with:

■ Insulin and diet
  – for Type 1 diabetes

■ Diet or diet and tablets (some people may need to take insulin injections) – for Type 2 diabetes.

Treatment must be maintained throughout life. This is necessary not only to avoid symptoms and the risk of coma, but also to minimise the risks of any later complications.

All forms of treatment require some modification to daily routines, and the performance of checks to ensure that treatment is effective. However, you should be able to achieve these with only minimal disturbance to your daily life.

From Chapter 2 onwards, this book explains in detail what has gone wrong in your type of diabetes. You will see how, with correct treatment, you should be able to maintain effective control.

Modern treatment allows the many thousands of people with diabetes to achieve complete, fruitful, healthy lives. Diabetes should not interfere with the vast majority of occupations. Many of the most successful people in the country not only have diabetes, but have fulfilled their ambitions in all walks of life. These include first-class sportsmen and women, politicians, actors, actresses, and successful members of all professions, people who bear witness to the fact that effective treatment can be combined with the highest achievement.

2

Type 2 (Non Insulin Dependent) Diabetes

If you are fully to understand your treatment you will require some more information about this type of diabetes. The objectives of this chapter are to help you appreciate

- How insulin controls glucose in the body.
- What has happened in your case.
- Why this may have occurred.
- The explanation of any symptoms you may have experienced.
- Why treatment is necessary, even if you have had no symptoms.
- Why treatment must be continued.

■ So what happens when you develop diabetes?

As stated in Chapter 1, diabetes is a disorder of glucose control in the body. Glucose levels in the blood are too high.

Where does blood glucose come from?

In the healthy individual, the level of blood glucose is kept within close limits. The major source of sugar is the food we eat. Blood glucose therefore goes up after a meal and reaches a peak about 60–90 minutes after eating. Then as time passes the level falls again.

To understand this further it is necessary to know some facts about the food you eat. This is made up of three basic types – carbohydrates, fats and proteins, all of which are essential for a balanced diet.

These three types of food are broken down by digestive processes in the intestine. The breakdown products of digestion are then absorbed into the bloodstream and carried to the individual body cells.

Carbohydrates, found in starchy foods such as bread and potatoes, are broken down and converted to glucose (sugar). Fat is converted to fatty acids. These fatty acids and the glucose are used to provide energy in the body. When protein is digested the resulting products (amino acids) are used to build cells and tissues. Any excess is converted to glucose.

Fats

**Carbohydrates
(starches
and sugars)**

Proteins

Fats, carbohydrates and proteins are essential

The main sources of blood glucose in food are therefore:

- Sweet things, eg extra sugar added to cereals, drinks containing sugar, sweets, jams, etc.
- Starchy foods, eg bread, potatoes, cereals, rice, pasta, chapattis, cassava, yam, etc.
- Other foods, eg protein may be converted to glucose.

If glucose intake is more than the body requires, the excess is stored in the liver. This store acts as a reserve for times of need, illness or injury. But once liver stores are filled, any excess is converted to fat. This is what happens if you eat too much over a long period. Too much of the other fuels (fats and proteins) will ultimately have the same effect – both blood glucose and body weight will increase.

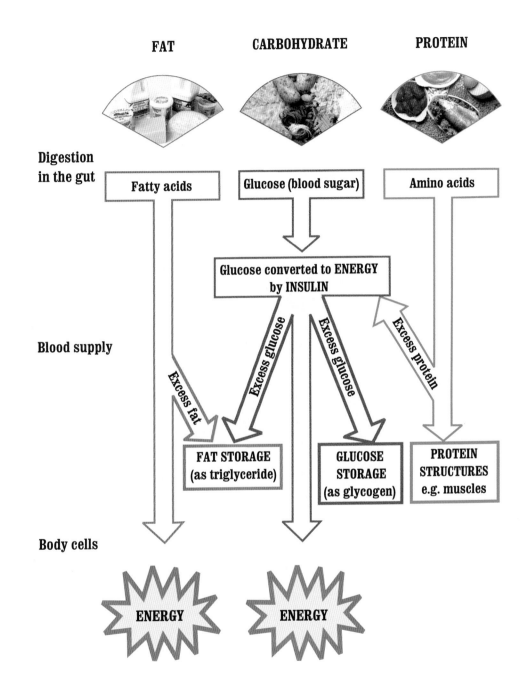

FAT   CARBOHYDRATE   PROTEIN

Digestion in the gut

Fatty acids   Glucose (blood sugar)   Amino acids

Glucose converted to ENERGY by INSULIN

Blood supply

Excess fat   Excess glucose   Excess glucose   Excess protein

FAT STORAGE (as triglyceride)   GLUCOSE STORAGE (as glycogen)   PROTEIN STRUCTURES e.g. muscles

Body cells

ENERGY   ENERGY

Normal metabolism. In the presence of insulin, glucose can be converted to energy

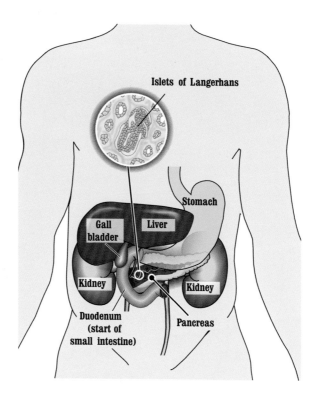

Islets of Langerhans

Stomach

Liver

Gall bladder

Kidney

Kidney

Duodenum (start of small intestine)

Pancreas

The pancreas is a large gland positioned behind the stomach. It contains many cells which produce insulin. These are collected in clusters called islets of Langerhans

The importance of insulin

Insulin is the key to the conversion of glucose to energy, or its storage. Insulin is produced by the pancreas, a gland situated at the back of the abdomen.

The pancreas is able to sense the level of blood glucose. As the glucose level rises, the pancreas will release more insulin into the circulation. This insulin reduces the blood glucose to the level at which it started. Thus, as the glucose level rises after a meal, the level of insulin increases as well. The level of insulin is therefore highest an hour or so following food, after which it falls back to its pre-meal level. The amount of insulin in the blood is lowest when you have not eaten, for example overnight.

When you are not eating, your blood glucose is kept steady and prevented from falling too low by a regular trickle of glucose into the blood from the body stores. This is finely balanced by a slow output of insulin. During exercise more glucose is used up, so in order to stop the level from falling too low, more glucose is released from stores. The insulin level is reduced.

At times of stress or injury more energy is required by the body and more glucose is produced, even if you are not eating. This glucose is then converted to energy by a slow release of insulin. The rise of blood glucose under these circumstances is controlled.

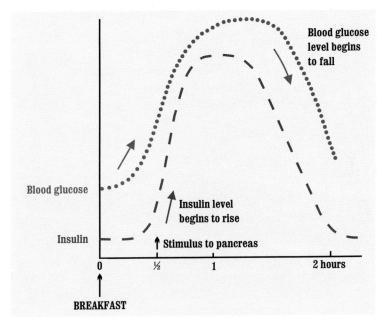

The control of blood glucose by insulin. Insulin released from the pancreas makes the blood glucose level fall. After 2–3 hours it returns to the same level as before the meal

What has gone wrong?

In your type of diabetes you are producing insulin, but not as much as you need. The situation is made worse if you are overweight, because the amount of fat in the body interferes with the action of the insulin. The rise in blood glucose after a meal is greater than normal and it does not return as quickly to its pre-meal level. When not eating, the blood glucose also tends to creep up as the energy stores release glucose in an uncontrolled way.

The effects of diabetes on blood glucose. In diabetes, insufficient insulin results in an excessively high blood glucose. It does not return to the normal level after eating

Blood glucose levels. When the glucose reaches a certain level, it spills over into the urine. This level is called the 'renal threshold'

As the blood glucose rises above normal, there comes a point when it begins to spill over into the urine (see lower illustration opposite). Usually, no glucose appears in the urine, so that when it is found it suggests that the blood glucose is too high. There are some people who spill glucose into the urine too easily, so that glucose appears in the urine but the blood glucose remains normal. This is called a 'low renal threshold'. In the case of diabetes, the presence of glucose in the urine means the blood glucose is too high.

■ Who gets diabetes? Why?

There are probably two factors that have contributed to the development of your diabetes:

1. You are not producing enough insulin.
2. The insulin that you are producing does not work as effectively as it did.

Type 2 diabetes occurs in various groups of individuals:

- ■ It occurs most commonly in people who are overweight. Fat tissue interferes with the action of insulin, so that overweight people need considerably more insulin. If, in addition, an overweight person has a lower than normal production of insulin (because of a defect in the pancreas), the supply of insulin will be insufficient to control the blood glucose. Overweight people tend to eat more than their body needs, and their food provides more glucose than can be processed by the available insulin. In most cases, the diabetes can be readily controlled by simply eating less and losing weight, thereby allowing the insulin to work more effectively.
- ■ This type of diabetes also occurs in people who are not overweight but who produce inadequate amounts of insulin.
- ■ Some people at times of stress show a tendency to be unable to produce enough insulin. This tendency may only become obvious at times when more glucose than normal is required. This may happen during an illness or after injury. It is important to point out that injury and illness are not believed to cause diabetes, but rather that they make it more obvious.
- ■ There is a strong hereditary element, and diabetes may be passed from generation to generation. However, it is not inevitable.
- ■ It is more common in some parts of the world, such as South America or Malta, than in others, such as Alaska.

- Certain ethnic groups in the UK, especially those from an African–Caribbean or Asian background, are more commonly affected.
- The frequency of diabetes increases with age.
- Sometimes it may occur temporarily in pregnancy. This is known as gestational diabetes.

Symptoms of high blood glucose

Glucose in the urine

As shown on page 14, one of the key features of a high blood glucose is spillage of glucose into the urine. This gives rise to three of the commonest symptoms of diabetes.

Passing large quantities of urine

In order to get rid of the excess glucose, more water is excreted by the kidneys. This results in the frequent passing of large volumes of urine, which may cause bedwetting in some children, or incontinence in the elderly.

Thirst

Because more water is leaving the body, the mouth becomes dry and thirst develops. This feeling may be very intense and disagreeable, and sometimes even talking and swallowing become difficult. Soft drinks which contain a lot of sugar should be avoided, as they actually increase the blood glucose, resulting in an even greater thirst.

Genital soreness

When a large quantity of glucose is passed in the urine, it tends to cause irritation around the genital area. The infection called thrush may develop. Thrush frequently causes itching of the vulva in women and, less often, itching of the penis in men.

Breakdown of body energy stores

Because a shortage of insulin means that the blood glucose cannot be converted into energy, energy must be provided from elsewhere. Consequently, there is a breakdown of fat and protein with the following results.

Weight loss

Diabetes is one of the commonest causes of weight loss. In most people with diabetes this occurs at the onset of the disorder, and it ranges from a few pounds to two to three stones. Appetite is commonly unaffected and may even be increased. Not everyone loses weight, so do not ignore other symptoms.

Tiredness and weakness

Tiredness, often accompanied by a sensation of weakness, is very common in uncontrolled diabetes. Some people find that they are more than usually prone to fall asleep at odd times, while others just feel they are growing old before their time. These symptoms can be readily reversed by treatment. Many people feel rejuvenated after treatment, even when they had previously been unaware of any abnormalities.

ALL THESE SYMPTOMS SHOULD DISAPPEAR SOON AFTER TREATMENT IS STARTED

If symptoms return, the glucose levels will have risen to too high a level and treatment will need to be adjusted.

Other effects of high blood glucose

Blurred vision

A high level of glucose in the body causes the lens of the eye to change slightly in shape, which may cause some blurring of vision. Sometimes this occurs after treatment has started. As the blood glucose returns to normal the lens may change shape again. These changes are only temporary, and within a few weeks the ability to focus should return to normal. Therefore, it is wise not to have your eyes tested for at least two months after proper stabilisation of your diabetes.

Excessive loss of fluid/diabetic coma

It is important to stress that in your type of diabetes, the so-called 'diabetic coma' (ketoacidosis), which results from an extremely high blood glucose level, does not occur. During any illness the blood glucose level is likely to rise. If you stop eating/drinking you may become short of fluid/dehydrated. This is especially likely if the illness is associated with vomiting.

Symptomless diabetes

Why treatment must be continued

Most people with diabetes are aware of symptoms when the blood glucose is very high. Others may be quite unaware of their condition. For instance, diabetes is often detected at a routine medical examination for insurance or employment purposes, or during an investigation of some quite unrelated illness.

- Very often symptoms disappear during the early stages of treatment, even though the blood glucose is still above normal.
- You will need to learn how to check that your glucose levels are not too high, even if you have no symptoms.
- If your tests are too high, your treatment may need to be increased.
- Either way, treatment must be continued whether you have symptoms or not.

Long-term effects of high blood glucose

If the blood glucose remains high for a period of years – even if it is not causing symptoms – it may cause harm. In particular, damage to the blood vessels, both the large vessels increasing the risk of heart attack and stroke – and the small blood vessels, which can affect the nerves, the back of the eye and the kidneys, may occur. Early, effective treatment of diabetes should prevent this damage from developing. Occasionally, some of these problems may be present when your diabetes is first discovered. However, treatment for your diabetes should stop them from developing further. Complications of diabetes are considered in more detail in Chapter 7.

3 Food and Physical Activity

This chapter describes the steps you need to take to control your diabetes and, in particular, gives details of the type of food you should eat.

There are two main aims of treatment:

1. Eliminate symptoms
2. Prevent late complications.

■ Eliminate symptoms

A high blood glucose level is largely responsible for your symptoms. The first aim of treatment is to reverse these by returning the blood glucose level to normal. Once treatment has started, although your diabetes has not been 'cured', your symptoms should disappear and should not recur if treatment is continued.

■ Prevent late complications

If a high blood glucose persists for many years, then the eyes, kidneys and small nerves to the feet may be damaged. Therefore, there is every reason to achieve acceptable blood glucose levels and, by keeping to your treatment, reduce the risk of these complications.

People with diabetes are two to five times more likely to develop problems with their major arteries, and this may lead to heart and leg trouble. This can be kept to a minimum by adjusting the diet in the way described below.

IT IS IMPORTANT THAT YOU CONTINUE WITH YOUR TREAT-
MENT, EVEN WHEN THE SYMPTOMS HAVE GONE, AND THAT
YOU UNDERGO REGULAR CHECKS TO ENSURE THAT YOUR
CONTROL IS BEING MAINTAINED.

■ The steps you need to take

Adjust what you eat

- Reduce your weight if necessary and try to keep it at an acceptable level. Most people with Type 2 diabetes are overweight. Being overweight makes the insulin you produce less efficient. The most important measure needed to control blood glucose levels is to reduce weight. Your aim should be to reach your target weight, when the insulin you produce will be able to maintain your blood glucose at an acceptable level. Losing a small amount of weight and keeping it off helps you to control blood glucose levels more easily.
- Eat regular meals based on starchy foods like bread, potatoes, rice, pasta, chapattis, yam, cassava and cereals.
- Reduce the amount of fat and fatty foods that you eat.
- Include more beans and pulses.
- Limit your sugar intake. It is important to avoid or reduce your intake of foods that lead to a rapid rise in blood glucose, particularly sweets, sweetened drinks and sugary puddings.
- Eat more fruit and vegetables. Aim for at least five servings a day.
- Use low fat dairy products on a regular basis.
- Increase your level of exercise or physical activity.
- Drink alcohol only in moderation.

All of these essential adjustments to your diet can be achieved fairly easily with time. You will still be able to enjoy everyday foods and delicious meals with your family and friends, as you did before you developed diabetes.

Other treatment measures

Unfortunately, with the passage of time your insulin levels may fall and adjusting what you eat may not control your blood glucose. Additional treatment is then necessary.

- Tablets. If the above measures prove inadequate, you may be advised to take some oral hypoglycaemic tablets. These are not, however, a substitute for diet.

■ Insulin treatment. Insulin injections are only required when all the above measures have proved ineffective.

This chapter describes the changes you may need to make in the type of foods you eat and your eating habits and how you might increase your level of physical activity. Tablet and insulin treatment are described in subsequent chapters.

■ What will the diet be like?

The diet for diabetes is not a special diet as such. It is, in fact, a healthy way of eating which is recommended for everyone. The purpose of this section is to help you make the best choice in the food that you eat.

■ Firstly, you may need to alter the sort of food you eat. Some foods like fat, salt and sugar should be limited, some like puddings and cakes eaten only in moderation, and some like fruit and vegetables may be eaten freely.

■ Secondly, you may need to adjust the amount of food you eat, especially if you are overweight.

Food plays a very important part in our lives, and therefore making changes to our diet can affect more than just meal times. Our eating patterns and the types of food we eat are often a lifelong habit. These habits are difficult to break, so do not expect to change your diet overnight. With the help of your local state registered dietitian, look realistically at what you are eating and decide what changes could easily be made. Tackle these first and then go on to the rest.

The basic components of food – a little theory

Our food is made up of three main groups – carbohydrate, protein and fat. They are all essential for a balanced diet. Most foods contain mixtures of one or more of these nutrients. For example, milk contains carbohydrate, protein and fat; eggs contain fat and protein and pastry is mainly fat and carbohydrate. In general vegetables and fruit contain little or no fat, while cheese, margarine and meat contain no carbohydrate.

FAT   CARBOHYDRATE   PROTEIN

Broken down by digestive processes

| Fatty acids and glycerol | Glucose and other simple sugars | Amino acids |

Absorbed into the bloodstream

| Provide energy or stored as energy reserves | Provide immediate energy | Used to build cells and tissues |

The three basic constituents of food

Carbohydrate

Carbohydrate is found in sugary and starchy foods.

Some typical carbohydrate-containing foods

All carbohydrates are broken down in the body to glucose (sugar) and so will cause the blood glucose level to rise. Choose starchy foods, eg bread, potatoes, breakfast cereals, rice, chapattis, cassava, yam and pasta, as the basis of all meals and snacks even if you are watching your weight. Eating starchy foods regularly helps blood glucose control.

However, very sugary foods, eg soft drinks and sweets, tend to be digested very quickly and cause a rapid and large increase in the blood glucose level. This increase may be short-lived and can produce swings from high to low. This may mean it is more difficult to control your diabetes.

Foods high in sugar

Protein

Foods high in animal protein include meat, milk, eggs, fish and dairy products. Some protein is essential in the diet, because it provides the building materials for the cells and tissues of the body. You will need to remember that foods high in animal protein also tend to be high in fat. Choose lean meats and bake, grill or steam rather than frying or cooking with extra fat or oil. Vegetable sources of protein, eg cereals and pulses, are a low fat alternative to animal protein and are also a good source of soluble fibre that is useful in helping to control blood glucose levels. Try to replace some of the animal protein in your diet with these foods.

These foods are all sources of protein

Fat

Only small quantities of fat are necessary for good health. Obvious sources of fat are butter, margarine, oil, lard and dripping; fatty meats and full-fat dairy products also contain fat. You should also watch out for the fat found in cakes, biscuits, snacks and pastries.

Foods high in fat

There are three types of fat:

- Saturated fats
- Monounsaturated fats
- Polyunsaturated fats.

They all contain the same amount of calories, but saturated fats particularly can raise blood cholesterol levels. Saturated fats are usually found in animal products, eg fatty meat, suet, lard, butter, cheese, milk and other dairy products.

Unsaturated fats should be used in preference to foods high in saturated fats. When choosing a cooking oil, select those which state on the label that they are high in monounsaturated or polyunsaturated fats. Monounsaturated fats are found in olive and rapeseed oil. They have also been shown to improve blood cholesterol levels. Oily fish, eg herring and mackerel, are particularly recommended. These contain a type of polyunsaturated fat which also helps keep cholesterol levels down. Try to eat this type of fish at least once a week.

It is not the amount of cholesterol in the food which affects blood cholesterol. Everybody has cholesterol in their blood. It forms an important part of cells and tissues. Unfortunately too much cholesterol can lead to a build up of fatty deposits in the arteries. Most cholesterol in the body is made from other food – especially saturated fat. Some foods are naturally high in cholesterol. Cutting these down has only a limited effect. The most benefit is achieved by eating less saturated fat. Cholesterol also rises as a person becomes overweight. Weight control will therefore help keep levels down.

It is important to remember that all types of fat are high in calories and only small quantities should be used. Whenever possible, try to choose monounsaturated or polyunsaturated fats in preference to saturated ones.

Fibre

Dietary fibre is a substance of plant origin which is not broken down in the human digestive system. It is good for helping to lower your blood glucose levels as well as helping to prevent constipation. High fibre foods also tend to be bulky, so they fill you up more quickly – this is especially important if you are trying to lose weight.

There are two types of fibre: insoluble and soluble. Insoluble fibre helps the prevention of constipation. Foods containing soluble fibre tend to have less effect on the rise in blood sugar and are therefore good for your blood glucose levels. Fruits and vegetables, and the outside coats of grains and cereals, all contain fibre.

Insoluble fibre is found in wheat bran, wholemeal flour, wholemeal bread, brown pasta and brown rice.

Foods that are high in soluble fibre are, for example, peas, beans, oats and lentils. They slow down the rise in blood glucose levels after a meal.

Foods high in soluble fibre

Remember that you do not have to eat wholemeal foods all the time, but try to include a variety of high-fibre choices across the day.

Here are some ways to increase your fibre intake:

- Add extra vegetables and pulses to soups and casseroles.
- Instead of white flour, use wholemeal flour or a mixture of half white and half wholemeal.
- Leave the skin on potatoes if using in recipe.
- Eat the skin of jacket and boiled potatoes.
- Add dried fruits to puddings, cakes and biscuits.
- Snack on fruit.
- Eat fruit-based puddings.
- Add pulses and pasta to salads.
- Add peas and/or sweetcorn to rice during cooking.
- Try a variety of breads, including wholemeal or granary.

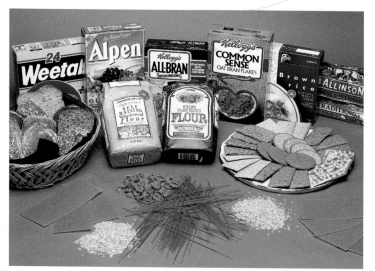

Foods high in insoluble fibre

Vitamins and minerals

There are many vitamins and minerals and they are all vital for good health. If you are eating the right balance of carbohydrate, protein and fat, sufficient quantities of vitamins and minerals should automatically be included in the diet. Supplements will not therefore be necessary.

■ Healthy eating – putting it into practice

Fruit and vegetables

Bread, other cereals and potatoes

Meat, fish and alternatives

Foods containing fat
Foods containing sugar

Milk and dairy foods

The balance of good health

In order to make the right choices it is easiest to think of meals as a whole. To do this, consider a plate of food. This is likely to consist of foods falling into five main groups:

- ■ Starchy carbohydrate, eg bread, potatoes, rice, pasta, cereals, chapattis, cassava, yam.
- ■ Fruit and vegetables.
- ■ Meat, poultry, fish, eggs or meat alternative (for example, beans and pulses).
- ■ Dairy foods – milk, cheese, yoghurts.
- ■ High fat and high sugar foods, eg jam, honey, butter, margarine, oils.

As explained in the previous section, you need to get a balance so that your plate contains a high proportion of starchy carbohydrate and fruit and vegetables, with small amounts of meat and fish (or alternatives) and milk and dairy foods. High fat and high sugar foods should be limited to small amounts.

Starchy carbohydrate

Examples of starchy carbohydrate foods

- Starchy carbohydrate foods are broken down to glucose for energy.
- Your diet must therefore contain enough carbohydrate to ensure a reasonable level of blood glucose in order to produce the fuel your body needs.
- Each of your meals should be based mainly on starchy foods, as the plate model shows. If you feel hungry between meals, choose snacks that contain starchy carbohydrate such as bread or rolls and cereals.
- You should not cut out foods containing carbohydrate. This would merely encourage your body to produce more glucose from its reserves, which would cause you to lose weight and become unwell. Starvation is no treatment for diabetes.
- Starchy foods which are high in fibre, especially soluble fibre, eg pasta, help slow down the rise in blood glucose further and are therefore good choices to include in your diet.

Fruit and vegetables

Fruit and vegetables are essential for a healthy diet

Fruit and vegetables should also be included in your diet in generous portions. A good guide is to include at least five servings of fruit or vegetables each day. They contain vitamins and fibre which help to even out blood glucose levels.

Remember, frozen and canned fruit in natural juice and vegetables are good alternatives to fresh. Try to have fruit and vegetables at each meal. Fruit is an ideal between-meal snack.

Meat, fish, eggs and pulses

Foods rich in protein

These foods provide the body with protein.

- To keep down the saturated fat in your diet, choose lean red meat and remove the skin from poultry. Grill, rather than fry, meat products including burgers and sausages.
- Aim to eat fish at least twice a week, one portion of which should be oily fish. White fish is lower in fat than meat. Oily fish such as tuna, salmon, sardines, mackerel and pilchards are fairly high in fat, but it is the kind of fat that helps to protect you from heart disease.
- Alternatives to meat such as peas, beans and lentils are a good source of protein but are low in fat. They also have a low glycaemic effect. Try replacing some of the meat in your diet with some of these.
- Soya products, such as tofu, and other vegetarian alternatives like Quorn are also low in fat and can be used to replace meat in certain recipes.

Milk and dairy foods

Full-fat milk and dairy foods contain a lot of saturated fat which can raise blood cholesterol. You can keep the fat down but still get the calcium you need by:

- Using semi-skimmed or skimmed milk
- Choosing low fat yoghurts
- Saving cream and cream products for special occasions
- Eating less cheese or using lower fat cheeses in place of full-fat varieties.

A daily intake of three servings will provide you with all the calcium that you need. A serving is one-third of a pint of milk, one pot of yoghurt or a piece of cheese the size of a small matchbox.

Fats and sugary foods

Reduced fat and fat-free products

Fats are very high in calories. If you are trying to avoid putting on weight you have to pay attention to the amount of fat in your diet. We suggest the following guidelines:

- Cut down on fatty foods and use less fat and oil in cooking
- Use monosaturated oil such as olive oil or rapeseed oil rather than saturated fat such as butter and lard
- Try not to have high fat snacks such as crisps, cakes and biscuits every day.

When you are first diagnosed you may have quite severe symptoms. To start with, therefore, you need to avoid sugary drinks and confectionery which cause a rapid rise in blood glucose levels. Sugary drinks can mostly be replaced with sugar-free alternatives – you can use a sweetener in place of sugar in hot drinks if you wish. Even these small changes can result in quite rapid improvement, with loss of symptoms and lowering of the blood sugar.

The aim is to produce a balanced diet (see plate model on page 29). It is perfectly acceptable to include some foods that are higher in sugar and fat, providing the total amount of food you eat is limited to ensure that you do lose weight when advised to do so and that you maintain your weight loss. Fatty and sugary foods should form only a small part of a balanced diet.

A wide range of low sugar and sugar-free products is available

The amount of sugar in a food does not alone reflect the amount of sugar in your blood. It is now recognised that the rise of blood sugar depends very much on the combination of foods within a meal and food intake across the day. You may have come across a term called the 'Glycaemic Index' (GI) applied to foods. This provides a comparison of how different foods containing carbohydrate affect blood glucose levels. Those with a high glycaemic index put up the blood sugar more than those with a low glycaemic index.

HIGH

Bread stuffing	Honey
Cheerios	Mashed potato
Choco Krispies	Morning Coffee biscuits
Cornchips	Parsnips
Cornflakes	Puffed Wheat
French baguette	Rice cakes
Glucose	Rice Krispies

MEDIUM

Arrowroot biscuits	Pineapple	Water biscuits
Couscous	Raisins	Water melon
Golden Grahams	Ryvita	Weetabix
Muesli	Shortbread	White bread
New potatoes	Shredded Wheat	Wholemeal bread
Pastry	Sustain	

LOW

All Bran	Digestive biscuits	Peanuts
Apple	Fruit bread	Porridge
Baked beans	Grapefruit	Pumpernickel bread
Banana	Grapes	Rich Tea biscuits
Black-eyed beans	Kidney beans	Rye bread
Brown rice	Lentils	Spaghetti
Buckwheat	Long grain rice	Special K
Bulgar wheat	Macaroni	Sultana Bran
Butter beans	Milk	Sweetcorn
Chick peas	Oat bran bread	Yoghurt
Crisps	Orange	

Examples of foods with high, medium and low glycaemic index

You cannot tell a low GI food just by looking at it – and GI is not just related to the fibre or sugar content of a food. The effect on blood glucose levels of a meal or snack is influenced by many things. The way in which a food is cooked and prepared, the combination of foods you eat with it and their fat and protein content, as well as other foods you have eaten that day can all have a bearing on its GI. It is not possible at the moment, therefore, to label all the foods we might eat according to their GI.

You do not need to exclude all foods with a high GI and eat only foods with a low GI. To apply the benefits of GI to your diet however, try to include low GI foods with each meal, which lowers the overall glycaemic effect of a meal. Low GI foods like fruit and vegetables, beans and pulses, pasta and oats form part of a well balanced diet anyway.

Finally, if you test your blood fairly regularly after meals you can gain some understanding of how food affects your blood sugar. Remember, food is not the only influence. Physical activity, diabetes medication, and illness can all affect blood glucose levels.

What are sweeteners?

There are two main types of sweetener: non-intense and intense sweeteners.

Non-intense sweeteners

These include fructose and polyols (like sorbitol, maltitol, mannitol, isomalt, xylitol). They are sometimes known as nutritive or bulk sweeteners.

Non-intense sweeteners are not recommended as sweeteners. This is because they offer no benefit over ordinary sugar to people with diabetes. They contain calories and carbohydrate and so can still cause blood glucose levels to rise. They also have a laxative effect. Foods that contain a significant amount of non-intense sweeteners have to be labelled with a warning 'Excessive consumption may produce laxative effects'. Non-intense sweeteners are commonly used in diabetic foods, tooth friendly sweets and some sugar-free confectionery.

Fructose (fruit sugar) is sometimes used in foods such as low fat yoghurts as an alternative to sugar. Diabetes UK does not feel that fructose in foods offers any special advantage over sugar to people with diabetes. Everyday foods that contain fructose can be eaten, but fructose is not recommended as a table top sweetener or for use in cooking.

Intense sweeteners

Intense sweeteners are also known as artificial sweeteners. There are four types that are most commonly used in food products in this country: aspartame (Nutrasweet™), saccharin, acesulfame potassium (acesulfame K) and cyclamates. The intense sweetener used in a food will always be in the ingredients listing – either the name or additive number.

Intense sweeteners are both carbohydrate and calorie free. They will not affect blood glucose levels. Because they are very intense only small amounts need to be used. These sweeteners are used widely in manufactured foods and are also available as tablet, liquid and granulated sweeteners for use at home. They can be used in drinks, on cereals and in certain puddings if you require extra sweetness.

Artificial sweeteners

Diabetic foods

There is no need to buy special 'diabetic' foods. They are unnecessary and offer no benefit over ordinary foods. They are usually expensive.

Salt

Eating too much salt can lead some people to develop high blood pressure. It is sensible to cut down on the amount of salt in your diet.

- ■ Reduce the amount of salt used in cooking and use less salt at the table.
- ■ Tinned, packaged and processed foods tend to be higher in salt, so eat less of these, but reduced salt versions of tinned or processed foods can be helpful.

Do calories matter?

Calories are a measure of the amount of energy provided by the food you eat. Their official name is actually kilocalories (kcal), but they are usually referred to simply as calories.

It is useful to think a little about calories, especially if you are trying to lose weight or avoid putting it on. To lose weight the body has to burn off more energy/calories than you eat. With the exception of some vegetables, eg lettuce, all food contains some calories. But weight for weight some foods contain very many more calories than others. For example, an average apple would provide 50 calories whereas the same weight of cheddar cheese would provide 400 calories. Generally speaking high-fat foods contain two and a half times the number of calories as the same weight of carbohydrate foods. When trying to lose weight, therefore, it is much easier and more effective to cut down on your fat intake.

Checking the label

What the terms mean

Energy: the amount of energy (calories) that a food provides. Look for the 'kcal' figure which means calories. To keep to a healthy weight, the energy we eat (found in calories) needs to balance with the amount of energy used in daily life.

Protein: protein is needed for growth and repair. Most adults eat more than enough protein so don't worry about this on the label.

Carbohydrate: the total carbohydrate in food, which includes sugars and starches. You should get most of the energy in your diet from starch. **Eat more**

"Of which sugars": the amount of the carbohydrate that is sugars – that's both natural and added sugars. **Eat less**

Fat: the total amount of fat in foods – polyunsaturated, monounsaturated and saturated fats. **Eat less**

"Of which saturates": the type of fat you need to particularly limit. **Eat less**

Fibre: fibre is important for a healthy bowel. **Eat more**

Sodium: indicates how much salt is in a food. **Eat less**

NUTRITION INFORMATION		
	per 100g	per 25g serving
ENERGY	1560 kj 367 kcal	390 kj 92 kcal
PROTEIN	7.3g	1.8g
CARBOHYDRATE of which sugars	82.7g 8.9g	20.7g 2.2g
FAT of which saturates	0.8g 0.3g	0.2g 0.1g
FIBRE	3.6g	0.9g
SODIUM	1.1g	0.3g

What the label tells you

Do the figures mean a lot or a little?

To judge whether a food contains a little or a lot of a nutrient, use the 'per 100g' figure for a snack food and the 'per serving' figure for a complete meal.

Energy: If you are overweight, you need to eat fewer calories and, if possible, increase the amount of activity you do to use up more calories.

Sugar: 10g or more of sugar is a lot. 2g or less of sugar is a little.

Fat: 20g or more of fat is a lot. 3g or less of fat is a little.

Saturates: 5g or more is a lot. 1g or less is a little.

Fibre: 3g or more is a lot. 0.5g or less is a little.

Sodium: 0.5g or more is a lot. 0.1g or less is a little.

Eating out

Most people enjoy eating out – whether at a restaurant, café or pub – and the odd meal that is higher in fat or sugar is fine. If you eat out more often, whether for social or work reasons, you need to be more careful about your food choices.

Having diabetes doesn't mean you can't try different types of food like Chinese, Indian, Thai or Italian. Different foods can have different effects on blood glucose levels but if you monitor your levels regularly you will gradually get to know the effects different foods have and be able to adjust your treatment for the next time.

Meals out are often richer than you would cook for yourself. If you eat out on a regular basis, these tips will help:

- Have an alcohol-free apéritif if you're going to have wine with your meal
- Avoid nibbling on peanuts or crisps before the meal – vegetable crudités, cocktail onions, gerkins or olives would be better
- Choose vegetable-based soup, melon, light salads or fish for starters. These are better choices than pâtés or deep-fried starters, like mushrooms or potato skins
- Instead of having meat, fish or poultry that has been fried or battered, or dishes that come with rich creamy or buttery sauces, ask for them to be grilled or chargrilled. Always remove visible fat from meat and skin from poultry
- Watch out for high fat dressings, mayonnaise and creamy dips. Ask for dressings, sauces and butter to be served separately. This way you have a choice of how much to add
- Fill up with plenty of salad, unbuttered vegetables and bread. If you've chosen a main course that does not contain much carbohydrate ask for extra bread or potatoes
- If you want a dessert, be tempted by a fruit-based pudding or sorbet rather than gâteaux, pastries or cheese and biscuits. And go easy on the cream!
- Finally especially if you're trying to lose weight, don't be shy – ask for small portions.

Alcohol

There is no reason why the moderate use of alcohol should not be a pleasant part of your life. However, you may want to think about what you drink and when.

Diabetes UK recommends the following
maximum intake of alcohol:

   3 units of alcohol a day for a man
   2 units of alcohol a day for a woman

where 1 unit =
   half a pint of ordinary beer, lager or cider
   1 pub measure of spirits
   1 glass of wine
   1 small glass of sherry
   1 measure of vermouth or aperitif

■ Take care if you are taking tablets to treat your diabetes.
   Alcohol may enhance their effects.

   1. Do not drink on an empty stomach.
   2. Do not substitute alcoholic drinks for your usual meal.

■ It is important to remember that all alcoholic drinks also contain
   calories and should therefore be limited if you are overweight.
■ Low sugar beers are best avoided as they are higher in alcohol than
   normal beers.
■ Low alcohol beers and lagers may be useful. However, low alcohol
   drinks, particularly alcohol-free wines, can be quite sugary. Remember
   they are not alcohol-free.
■ Always use low calorie/sugar-free mixers and be careful of home measures.
■ Never drink and drive.

Watching your weight

Most people (approximately 80 per cent) with your type of diabetes are
overweight.

Weight loss is the most important measure needed to control blood glucose levels. It
is very difficult to control your diabetes if you remain significantly overweight,
and your tablets will not work as effectively as they could. There is also an increased
risk of conditions such as heart disease, high blood pressure and arthritis.

Some people can lose weight more quickly than others, but no one finds it easy.
You have to look honestly at what you are actually eating and try to pinpoint
areas where you could cut down. Are you eating lots of fatty foods, such as fatty

meats, lots of butter, crisps, nuts, pastries and pies? Are you eating late at night? Could you be making better use of low-calorie or high-fibre foods?

The type of diet you choose must be nutritionally balanced. Miracle diets or very low calorie diets can be tempting, but they do not have long-term benefits.

People vary in the way they wish to approach their weight reduction diet. Some prefer to follow general guidelines. They feel sufficiently in control not to have to plan meals strictly in advance and consider themselves capable of selecting the best choice at the time. Others are more comfortable if they plan in advance and determine exactly what each meal should contain.

Body Mass Index (BMI)

Your weight is often calculated as BMI which expresses adult weight in relation to height. From this you will be advised if you need to lose weight to help control your diabetes. Your GP will record your BMI in your notes.

To calculate your BMI: $$BMI = \frac{weight\ (kg)}{height\ (m)^2}$$

A BMI of 20–25 is classed as a healthy weight (see the chart above). You do not need to lose weight.

A BMI of 25–30 is classed as overweight. The health risks for those in this range are associated with the extra weight being carried around your middle.

A BMI greater than 30 is associated with significantly increased health risks.

Hints on weight control

- Set yourself a realistic target. Any weight loss, if it is kept off, is better than none.
- If you are very heavy do not aim to achieve a normal weight. A weight loss of one and a half stones (10 kg) has significant benefits to health.
- Losing weight takes time. Eating sensibly and aiming to lose weight slowly will help maintain good blood glucose control. Weight which is lost at a rate of 0.5–1 kg (1–2.2 lbs) a week is more likely to stay off.
- Only weigh yourself once a week and at the same time of day. Because your weight fluctuates naturally from day to day, you may become disheartened if you weigh yourself too often.
- Diet and exercise together is the best way to lose weight and to keep it off.
- Never miss a meal or you will be extremely hungry at the next one and may then find it difficult to stick to your diet. You will lose weight more easily if you eat more regular meals, rather than saving up your calories for a large supper at the end of the day.
- Avoid slimming products. They may seem like an easy option but if you lose weight quickly you are likely to return to your old weight once you start eating normally again.
- Avoid so-called diabetic foods. Most are high in calories and fat.
- You may find it useful to plan your meals the day before. If you know what you are going to eat at each meal, then you will not be tempted to take the first thing you see in the cupboard.
- Always try to sit down to eat a meal. It is surprising how much you can eat without noticing it when you are on the move!
- Do not prepare too much food. If there are two of you in the family, prepare meals for two, not four. You will be tempted by the leftovers, as no one likes to see food thrown away.

■ Have plenty of low calorie foods (eg salads and vegetables) on hand for when hunger strikes.

■ Never shop when you are hungry, or you will be tempted to buy more. It may help to make a shopping list; if you keep to it, you will be less likely to stray into the supermarket aisles where they display the cakes and sweets.

■ If you have to buy sweets and crisps for your family, try to avoid bulk buying. If you have children who are fond of chocolate, buy them just one bar at a time, rather than a packet containing several bars. Having the extra bars around is simply putting temptation in your way! If possible, persuade your family to buy their own treats and to eat them when you are not around.

■ Finally, ask your family doctor to refer you to a state registered dietitian. A dietitian can recommend a calorie intake and eating plan that suits your lifestyle, is medically safe and which contains the correct balance of nutrients.

■ Exercise – part of your treatment

Regular physical activity has many beneficial effects.

■ It improves the efficiency of your insulin.
■ It reduces both glucose and fat levels in the blood by burning off excess food intake.
■ It helps you to control your weight.
■ It will improve your blood pressure.
■ It improves the circulation to heart and limbs.
■ It will make you more relaxed.
■ It should be enjoyable!
■ It helps you remain more active as you get older.

Exercise is strongly recommended, therefore, to help with your treatment.

How much exercise?

To obtain the benefits, exercise needs to be performed regularly, preferably on a daily basis. It is recommended that you take 30 minutes of brisk exercise five times a week. You need to build into your daily life a routine to allow this. It is not wise to engage in occasional sudden bursts of exercise – this may do you more harm than good.

What sort of exercise?

There are two types of exercise:

- Energetic exercise which will make you sweaty, short of breath and keep you moving for 20 minutes or more, eg running, brisk hill climbing, biking.
- Steady sustained exercise which does not cause shortage of breath, eg walking, playing golf, cycling on the flat, gardening.

Your choice will depend very much on your existing exercise habits. If you can work up to the point of getting short of breath on a regular basis, this is better for you. You must get into training to do this, ie increase your regular exercise gradually over several weeks (like an athlete training for a race).

If you take very little exercise normally (ie only gentle housework, driving to work or the shops), consider trying to achieve a 30–60 minutes' walk per day or every other day over a period of six to eight weeks. Start with 10 minutes, increasing by 5–10 minutes per day every week. Alternatively, you could take up regular swimming: start with 10 minutes in the pool per day and work up to regular swimming of a number of lengths, gradually increasing the number.

If you already take some regular exercise, such as golf once or twice a week, increase this by adding, again relatively gradually, an hour a day of brisker walking, gardening or cycling. Consider taking up more energetic physical activity so that you get a bit short of breath on a fairly regular basis.

Keep fit by doing something that you enjoy

Some people who develop diabetes are already quite elderly and may be relatively disabled, for example by arthritis. It is still possible to take some exercise. Even those who have difficulty walking, perhaps due to problems with knees or hips, can start regular exercise sitting in a chair. Discuss with your doctor how you can get an exercise plan involving arm swinging, forward side bends, leg swinging or calf and ankle exercises.

If you already have problems with the circulation to your legs, ie you get pain in the calves on walking, don't be put off. Walk to the point of pain – note how far you have got, stop and let the pain subside – increasing the number of times you do this every day. Gradually you will find the distance you go improves. Keep this going and you will feel the benefit.

More advice can be obtained from your local Sports Centre or from the Look after Yourself Project Centre (Christ Church College, Canterbury, Kent CT1 1QU).

Choose exercise that:

- You enjoy
- Makes you feel good
- You can do regularly for 20–30 minutes daily
- You can fit into your everyday routine
- You can do near or in your home
- Does not depend on the weather
- Suits your particular fitness needs.

Finally, exercise only helps if you keep doing it regularly.

■ Summary

- If you are overweight try very hard to lose weight.
- Eat regular meals and snacks if needed, including plenty of starchy carbohydrate foods (eg bread, potatoes, rice, pasta and cereals).
- Eat plenty of high-fibre foods, including fruit and vegetables.
- Watch your fat intake and avoid eating lots of fat and fatty foods.
- Control your sugar intake by restricting your intake of sweet and sugary foods.
- Use salt in moderation.
- Take care with alcohol.
- Increase the amount of exercise you take.

4 Tablet Treatment

Sometimes treatment with diet alone is not effective. In this case you may need to take tablets in conjunction with your diet. This chapter describes the tablets, how and when you should take them, and answers questions you may have about side-effects and alteration of the dose.

■ Which tablets?

There are five main types of tablets.

1. Sulphonylureas – these tablets stimulate you to produce more insulin. They are usually prescribed for those of normal weight who may be experiencing lack of insulin.
2. Biguanide type, eg metformin – these tablets help your insulin to work more efficiently. They are usually prescribed if you are overweight.
3. Glitazones – these tablets have only recently been introduced. They would appear to be particularly helpful in reducing the resistance to insulin action which is common in your type of diabetes.
4. Drugs to delay the absorption of carbohydrate, eg acarbose – these are usually tried when other agents have not worked.
5. Prandial glucose regulators – these are similar to sulphonylureas, but are only taken with food.

■ Some important questions about tablet treatment

When should tablets be taken?

- ■ Sulphonylurea type tablets should normally be taken once or twice a day with food.
- ■ Biguanides should be taken once or twice a day with or after meals.
- ■ Glitazones should be taken once a day, irrespective of meal times.
- ■ Acarbose must be taken one to three times daily with the first mouthful of a meal.
- ■ Prandial glucose regulators are taken before each meal.

Can I relax my diet?

No. Unfortunately tablets will only work in addition to your diet. If you relax your diet, good control is most unlikely.

Am I at risk until my blood glucose returns to normal?

Initially, your treatment with diet, or with a combination of diet and tablets, will take a few weeks to return your blood glucose to a normal level. During this period, however, you will come to no harm. The long-term complications of diabetes, which affect the eyes, kidneys, circulation and nerves, take many years to develop.

What happens if the tablets do not work?

If your blood glucose remains high, in spite of taking tablets, and you are carefully following your diet, your doctor may initially recommend several different types of tablets. If these do not work, your doctor may recommend insulin. Most instances of difficulty with control are due to a failure to follow the diet.

Can the blood glucose go too low?

Yes. This is called hypoglycaemia and can occur with sulphonylurea tablets and prandial glucose regulators but not with diet alone. It does not occur after glitazones, metformin or acarbose. It is usually easily recognised, as you will generally feel sweaty, hungry and possibly faint. In particular, it may occur if you have not eaten for some time. The common symptoms of hypoglycaemia include:

- Trembling
- Sweating
- Tingling around the mouth
- Palpitations of the heart, and then
  - Difficulty in concentration
  - Confusion
  - Muzziness
  - Faintness
  - Headache
  - Blurring of vision
  - Unsteadiness
  - Irritability, bad temper
  - Unusual lack of cooperation.

If my blood glucose goes too low, what should I do?

Immediately have something to eat or drink that contains quickly released sugar, eg sweets, glucose tablets, a sugary drink – ordinary Lucozade or ordinary lemonade – or some fruit juice. Follow with a meal if it is due, or a starchy snack such as a biscuit, toast or cereal. Sometimes the symptoms come back an hour or so later. If this happens, you should have some more to eat. If the symptoms recur on more than one day, or if they do not disappear after you have eaten something, then you will need to see your doctor. You should tell your doctor anyway on your next visit. The dosage of the tablets may need adjusting.

Can tablets cause other side-effects?

Side-effects are rare.

The sulphonylurea tablets cause no serious ill effects in the many thousands of people who take them. Slight swelling of the ankles may be noted in the early stages of treatment, and weight gain of a few pounds can occur. Skin rashes occur very occasionally.

Diarrhoea or abdominal pains are not uncommon at the start of treatment with metformin but usually wear off. If they persist, stop the metformin tablets and consult your doctor. With acarbose flatulence is common.

Prandial glucose regulators may cause abdominal pain, diarrhoea, constipation, nausea, vomiting and hypersensitivity reactions such as rashes.

Headaches, some increase in weight, oedema (fluid accumulation such as swelling in legs and ankles), anaemia and stomach disturbances may occur with glitazones.

Can I drive with tablet treatment?

Yes (but see section on driving, page 66). If you do have any odd feelings that might be due to hypoglycaemia be very careful. The symptoms may interfere with concentration and ability to drive. Stop immediately and have something to eat. You should always carry some biscuits or something similar in the car, just in case. Do not start to drive again until you feel better. Do not drive at all if you feel unwell.

Are there any other alternative treatments?

A number of herbal remedies have been tried. None are of proven benefit. Some may have marginal effects on blood glucose. Do let your doctor know if you plan to or are already taking any of these products, and do not stop taking your prescribed tablets.

■ Summary

- ■ Tablet treatment is used when changes in the diet provide insufficient control.
- ■ Tablets have very few side-effects and in most people none at all.
- ■ Metformin tablets can cause stomach disturbance, and acarbose flatulence, but these can often be avoided by starting on a low dose.
- ■ Occasionally, low blood glucose levels can occur – if you suspect this, have something to eat straight away.

5 Is Your Treatment Effective?

The aim of diabetes treatment is to return and keep your blood glucose within normal limits.

Unfortunately, how you feel is not a reliable guide to the level of your blood glucose. Symptoms, such as thirst, weight loss and passing large amounts of urine, appear only if the diabetes is badly out of control. Even with moderately high levels of blood glucose – the sorts of levels which can, over a period of years, lead to serious complications – you may have no symptoms. Therefore, it is important to ensure that your diabetes control is being maintained at an acceptable level. This chapter describes simple tests which enable you to check that your treatment is effective.

■ Blood tests versus urine tests

Blood glucose levels can be assessed either directly by means of blood tests, or indirectly by urine tests. Urine tests have the advantage that they are painless. Also, because they are much simpler to perform, they can easily be carried out at home. Therefore, for many of those with Type 2 (non insulin dependent) diabetes, regular urine testing will provide an effective guide to blood glucose levels.

However, for some people, urine tests can be misleading, because they fail to record high levels when they should and cannot show if your blood glucose level is low. Furthermore, for urine tests to be positive the blood glucose levels may need to be high for quite a while. Fairly short peaks after a meal may not show in the urine. If the tests performed when you attend your clinic or doctor reveal that your urine tests are not telling you all that they should, you will be advised to perform blood tests. In addition, some people prefer to use blood tests because they are unhappy about handling urine, although it is usually perfectly sterile and clean.

The techniques available for self blood glucose testing are now much easier and an increasing number of people prefer this method. Blood tests require only a single drop of blood, which you can obtain by pricking your finger. The test usually takes less than a couple of minutes to do, but must be carried out carefully to ensure an accurate result.

■ Urine tests

How urine tests work and their interpretation

When the blood glucose rises, a point is reached at which glucose starts to leak into the urine. In the majority of people this will happen whenever the blood glucose is too high, usually above about 10 mmol/l. Therefore, if the blood glucose has exceeded this threshold level since you last passed urine, a test for glucose in the urine will be positive. If the blood glucose is below this level, the urine tests will be negative.

What should you aim for?

Normally, the blood glucose should not rise above a certain level (9–10 mmol/l). Therefore, if you are testing blood, you will be encouraged to keep your levels below 10 mmol/l; if testing urine it should be free of glucose.

■ Overall assessment of your blood glucose

You may discover that your tests are not within an acceptable range all the time. As mentioned elsewhere, occasional high tests do not matter. You may also find that tests taken before meals may be normal or even low, but that those after meals, especially breakfast, may be high. Does this matter? Not necessarily. What is important is that the average blood glucose over weeks or months is acceptable.

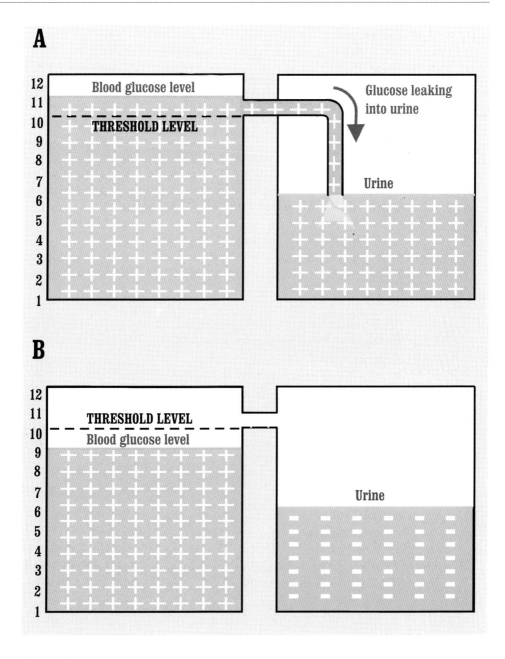

How urine tests work

Fortunately a test can and should be performed when you visit the doctor or clinic which tells you the answer. This is called the Haemoglobin A_{1c} (HbA_{1c}) test (or less commonly the fructosamine test). This measures the glucose level over the previous 6–12 weeks. If this is too high then adjustment of your treatment may be necessary. Those who are only doing urine tests may be advised to do blood tests as well if this test is higher than desirable.

Always ask for the result of the test when you see your doctor or nurse.

What should you do if the tests are high?

An occasional reading out of the normal range is acceptable. Sometimes a high reading is inexplicable. Usually high readings can be related to extra stress, less exercise, eating more than normal, or perhaps forgetting your diabetes tablets.

You should not be surprised to get high readings if you are feeling ill. Illness increases the blood glucose levels and, as with high urine tests, repeated high blood tests may indicate the need for a temporary change in treatment.

The long-term test helps to show whether the unusually high tests are too frequent. If this is normal then high tests are sufficiently infrequent not to matter. If raised it suggests the overall level is not entirely satisfactory.

How often should you do tests?

To start with you will be asked to test several times a day, because this will help you to understand what causes the blood glucose to rise. As your urine tests become negative, ie as your blood glucose returns to normal, two or three tests a week may be sufficient to reassure you that all remains well. Do not give up testing altogether just because you have reached the point where all the tests are normal. Things can change without you noticing. Stress and illness can also increase your blood glucose. Therefore, you would be wise to test at least four times a day during any illness – even a cold or flu – in order to discover whether your treatment is still effective.

Testing allows you to see how your diabetes is controlled, helping you to make changes to your diet and lifestyle. If your long-term test result is raised you may need to test more often.

When should you test?

Once treatment has begun to take effect, you will only wish to know if at any time the blood glucose is unusually high. Therefore, you should perform your urine test two hours after a main meal, since it is at this time that your blood glucose will be at its highest, and before breakfast to find out if your sugar is running high overnight. However, if you feel unwell, it is wise to test several times a day.

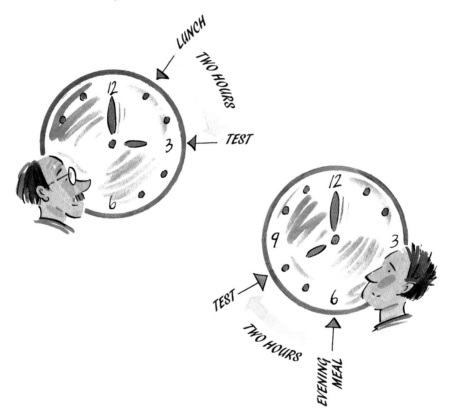

Keep a record of your tests

Isolated tests of the urine are of little value, but a regular record gives a much better idea of the level of control being achieved. Such a record will be of particular value when you attend your doctor or clinic for your regular medical check-up. Each test should be recorded on a chart or in a book (see overleaf).

Date \ Time	8 am	2.30 pm	6 pm	10 pm	Remarks:
Mon	nil				
Tues	nil				
Wed		++			After meal
Thu	nil				
Fri				nil	
Sat					
Sun	+++				Heavy meal night before

(Urine glucose column heading spans 8 am, 2.30 pm, 6 pm, 10 pm)

Keep a record of your urine tests

How are urine tests performed?

There are various urine tests available, all quite satisfactory. The main brands are Diastix and Diabur-Test 5000 (test strips). All the tests involve placing test strips in urine and observing a colour change. You should be shown how to test your urine when you first develop diabetes. If you have any doubts as to whether you are doing it correctly, check with your doctor or clinic. Urine tests depend on a colour change, so if you cannot see well, or if you are colour blind, you may not be able to detect the change and the tests may need to be done for you.

Urine test kits

■ Blood tests

Blood testing technique

Blood tests should be performed carefully. It is easy to get an inaccurate result if the correct technique is not followed. The doctor or nurse should instruct you in the proper procedure and show you how to read the results of your blood tests. Many people read the results by matching the change in colour of the strip against a colour chart on the strip container. Most people now buy a blood glucose meter (not available on prescription) which will measure the blood glucose automatically. Although a meter gives you a more precise reading, it does not make the test any more accurate. You still need to carry out the technique carefully.

If you can 'read' the strip by comparing it with the chart, there is no need to purchase a meter. Some meters use strips which cannot be read by eye. If you do decide to purchase a meter there are many to choose from, which you will find advertised in *Balance*, the Diabetes UK's magazine.

As with urine tests, blood tests are best performed before breakfast and one to two hours after a meal or, if you are unwell, before each meal. You might also want to test if you feel you are going hypo. If you write the results down, you can discuss their meaning with your doctor (see overleaf).

Availability of testing strips

Materials for urine or blood testing are available on prescription. Meters have to be purchased at prices from £25 to £60 – offers are sometimes available. Be sure to check the expiry dates of your testing strips.

| Month **APRIL** | | Test time | | | | | | | Comments |
Day	Date	Before breakfast	After breakfast	Before lunch	After lunch	Before dinner	Evening	Before bed	Medication, illness, etc.
MON	1	6.0							Diabetes tablet, 2 daily
TUES	2		11.0						
WED	3								
THURS	4				12.0				
FRI	5								
SAT	6						7.0		
SUN	7	4.0							
	8								
	9								
	10								
	11								
	12								
	13								
	14								
	15								
	16								

Blood tests – recording the test results. Always record your test using a record diary such as this

■ Regular weighing

Your weight is likely to be a major indication of success if you are being treated with diet alone. You will be advised of the most appropriate weight for your height, and be given a target to aim for if you are overweight. If your weight is normal, occasional weight checks are also important as an increase may well cause a deterioration in your diabetes control.

Unexpected loss of weight may indicate a change in your diabetes control, so if this happens do discuss it with your doctor.

■ When diabetes goes out of control

Factors leading to loss of control

In certain circumstances diabetes may go out of control unexpectedly. These are the five most common causes of loss of control.

1. The development of an acute infection

- Urinary infection
- Large boils, carbuncles, or abscesses
- Severe chest infection
- More seriously – gastroenteritis associated with vomiting
- Other physical illnesses, eg fractured limbs or operations.

2. After starting certain medications

- Especially steroids (prednisolone, cortisone)
- Sometimes certain water tablets (diuretics) used in the treatment of high blood pressure and heart disease.

3. Stressful situations

When people with diabetes are worried or anxious, they may find that their diabetes becomes more difficult to control.

4. Failure to respond to tablets

In some people with diabetes, the tablets may lose their effect after a period of satisfactory control. Changing to a different tablet may correct the situation, but some people may need to be re-stabilised with insulin.

5. Difficulty in following the advised treatment

People with diabetes who abandon their diet, forget or stop taking their tablets, or both, will almost certainly become badly controlled, although the deterioration may be quite a gradual process.

What you should do

In any of these situations, the blood glucose may rise and large amounts of glucose may be passed in the urine. Most illnesses, such as flu and colds, are of short duration and have no significant long-term effects, though the blood glucose, and hence blood glucose tests, may show increases for a day or so. An occasional dietary indiscretion may also show itself in a similar way. If, however, the urine tests become positive for glucose for more than a couple of days or your blood tests are consistently 10 mmol or more, you may need additional treatment and you should contact a member of your diabetes care team.

Vomiting and severe diarrhoea are, however, of greater significance, because they may cause the loss of a substantial amount of fluid and consequently an increased thirst. Although a person with Type 2 diabetes does not develop ketoacidosis (diabetic coma), the salt balance in the blood may become disturbed.

You must consult your family doctor if:

■ Despite plenty of fluid to drink, you still feel thirsty and unwell, and
■ All your urine tests are positive, or
■ Your blood tests are more than 15 mmol/l.

Very occasionally, your doctor may decide you need admission to hospital, so that:

■ If you have lost a large quantity of fluid this can be replaced by intravenous drip, and
■ Insulin can be given as required, at least temporarily.

■ Summary

■ Some regular checks are essential to see if your treatment is working.
■ You should perform these checks at least twice a week, and more often if you wish to, especially if you diabetes is not under control or you are ill.
■ Urine tests may be quite satisfactory for many people with your type of diabetes.
■ Some may prefer blood testing, which is quite easy to perform.
■ Blood tests are essential for some people, because their urine tests can give misleading information.
■ You should have a long-term blood test (HbA_{1c}) from time to time, to check that your own tests are accurate.
■ People on tablets which can cause low blood sugars should discuss blood testing with their doctor.

6 Insulin Treatment

Sometimes, despite sticking to your diet and receiving additional treatment with tablets, your glucose levels may continue to be too high. If this happens it is possible that your doctor will recommend insulin treatment. Although there is quite a lot to learn when starting insulin injections, this chapter summarises what you can expect. More detailed information is provided in the book *Living with Diabetes: The Diabetes UK Guide for those Treated with Insulin*, which is also published by John Wiley & Sons on behalf of Diabetes UK.

It should be stressed that this is not the same as Type 1 or insulin dependent diabetes. People with Type 1 diabetes have stopped producing insulin altogether. In your case it may be that you are still producing insulin, but in insufficient quantities.

Fortunately, insulin treatment for people with your type of diabetes is rather easier than for people with Type 1 diabetes who are producing no insulin at all. Although you are still producing insulin, the amount may be insufficient to prevent the blood glucose from remaining at too high a level. The decision to start insulin will usually only be taken when your doctor is sure the diet and tablet treatment has not worked.

■ Why injections?

Unfortunately, if insulin is taken by mouth it is simply digested and destroyed before it gets properly into the body. For this reason it has to be given by injection. You will therefore have to learn to give the injections yourself. This, however, is much easier than you might think. Most people find that it hurts very little.

■ Insulin treatment

Overall aims

The main purpose of treatment with injections is to copy the normal situation, ie to provide levels of insulin in the blood similar to those found in people whose insulin production is working correctly. The graph on page 13 shows how insulin is normally released into the blood after meals. The level rises as the glucose level rises, and falls again as the effect of the meal wears off. The blood glucose returns to normal under the influence of the insulin.

The aim, therefore, is to provide a peak of insulin at the times when the blood glucose is highest. It takes a little while for the insulin to get from the injection site into the circulation. This usually means giving it 30 minutes or

so before a meal. The injections usually have to be given twice a day. Some people find it easier to have smaller, more frequent injections with a larger injection at night. The aim will be to find the right combination to meet your needs.

Injecting insulin is much easier and less painful than you might think

What happens if you have too much insulin?

The blood glucose will fall too low if too large a dose of insulin is given. This is a condition known as hypoglycaemia or, for short, a 'hypo'. It is also sometimes referred to as an 'insulin reaction', or just a 'reaction'. When this happens a number of symptoms occur. These include sweating, fainting, hunger, or palpitations. You will be taught to recognise the symptoms and you should take sugar or a sugary drink as soon as you feel them coming on. It usually only takes a few minutes before you feel normal again. Very rarely, if the symptoms are not recognised, you may become unconscious. Eventually you will come round, as the body restores the glucose level to normal and the insulin effect wears off. No harm should come to you, but prevention is better than cure. If you eat regular meals and check your blood glucose, you should be able to avoid hypos fairly easily.

Testing

Up until now you may have only used urine testing. This, however, will only tell you how high the glucose has been. Urine tests give you no indication of the low blood glucose levels which might lead to hypoglycaemia. With insulin treatment the blood glucose changes more quickly and to a greater extent than with diet or tablets. In the first instance you will need to test to find out the correct doses and frequency of injections, and the right balance between injections and meals. You will want to make adjustments in order to fit your insulin treatment into your daily life without too many changes. For this reason it is recommended that blood testing is performed, which will give you a much more accurate picture of what is going on. Further details of urine and blood tests are given in Chapter 5.

Some questions about insulin treatment

Is insulin treatment for ever?

Usually, yes. Once it has been decided that you are not producing enough insulin to remain well, the insulin injections will probably need to be continued permanently. Sometimes, however, insulin treatment may be used as a temporary measure when some other illness makes your diabetes more difficult to control than usual. For example, this might happen after a heart attack, an operation, or a serious infection. The insulin will then be stopped as you recover.

During pregnancy, insulin may be started to ensure perfect control while you are carrying the baby. It will usually be discontinued when your baby is born.

Does the dose keep on going up?

No. Once you have worked out your usual daily dose, this will not increase to any major degree. However, your blood glucose may vary according to what you do or eat. Day-by-day variation is common. You may therefore have to make small adjustments on a day-to-day basis to fit in with your lifestyle. You may need an increased dose if you develop another illness, but these increases are usually temporary.

Does the diet need adjusting?

You cannot relax your diet completely once you have started insulin. If you do, your weight will increase and the insulin will work less efficiently. There-fore, you will have to continue to watch your total calorie intake. Sugar and sweet sugary foods are still not advisable as they will produce very rapid increases of blood glucose. These are difficult to correct without large and frequent doses of insulin, which will increase the risk of hypoglycaemia. It is important to ensure that your meals are taken regularly. If you miss meals after taking your insulin, the risk of too low a blood glucose (hypoglycaemia) is high. It may also be advisable to have a snack last thing at night.

Insulin injections and normal daily life

You should be able to undertake normal sporting activities, work (including shift working), physical exercise, etc. You may, however, have to make some adjustments to the carbohydrate you eat and to your insulin doses. Most people quickly learn how to do this, with the help of the clinic if necessary.

Driving

Particular care is needed while driving. This is to prevent hypoglycaemia, which could cause an accident.

- Always test yourself before a journey.
- Don't drive for too long without a meal or snack.
- Always carry sugar with you in case you get any of the symptoms of hypoglycaemia.

- Always stop if you do get any such symptoms.
- You must inform the DVLA and your insurance company that you have started insulin injections (see pages 89 and 91).

How will taking insulin affect my work?

Most people with diabetes can continue with their normal work

Most people are able to continue with their normal work. Unfortunately, certain jobs are closed to those taking insulin, including joining the armed services, flying, or working at sea. Exceptions may be made for some jobs, however, for serving members who have to start injections after treatment with diet and tablets. Driving public service vehicles, trains, or heavy goods vehicles (greater than 3.5 tonnes – but see page 111), and flying aircraft are normally not allowed. For most jobs, though, there should be no problems. If, however, you do a job in which temporary loss of consciousness might cause you or others to be in danger, then you need to discuss this with your doctor. Diabetes UK may also be able to help you to state your case to your employer.

More information

If you do have to start insulin treatment you will require more information. As mentioned previously, this is provided in the book *Living with Diabetes: The Diabetes UK Guide for those Treated with Insulin*, which is also published by John Wiley & Sons, Ltd on behalf of Diabetes UK.

■ Summary

- ■ Insulin treatment may be necessary for some people with your type of diabetes.
- ■ This will only be necessary if diet, or diet and tablet treatment, is not controlling your diabetes well enough.
- ■ Insulin is easier to give than most people expect, but does have to be given by injection.
- ■ Full instructions will be provided to make this as easy for you as possible.

7 The Long-Term Effects of Diabetes and Your General Health

This chapter describes the possible long-term effects of diabetes, how they may affect you, and the sort of treatment that can be given. An outline is also provided of the type of medical care and supervision you should expect.

Treatment of diabetes very rapidly restores health to normal. The symptoms disappear quite quickly and any loss of weight or of energy soon returns to normal.

After many years of diabetes, however, some of the body's tissues may be damaged. The eyes, kidneys, some nerves (mainly those to the feet), and the blood vessels are most susceptible. These problems are likely to develop only after many years of high blood glucose levels. The risk of these is much reduced if you can keep good control of your glucose levels. Many people are completely spared these problems and, even after more than 40 years of diabetes, show no trace of any complications.

■ Arterial disease and high blood pressure

Degeneration or hardening and narrowing of the arteries (blood vessels) are normal consequences of ageing. With diabetes, however, these are more likely. This may cause poor circulation in the feet and legs and can contribute to heart attack or stroke.

Particular attention to these aspects of your health can help minimise these serious problems.

High blood pressure

High blood pressure (hypertension) is more common in people with diabetes. We now recognise that it is particularly important for this to be treated, especially in those with diabetes. This will reduce the risk of heart attack or stroke. Indeed, the standards set for treatment of blood pressure for those with diabetes are now rather more strict than for those without.

There are a wide range of tablets which can be used and it is uncommon to fail to find a tablet or combination of tablets which cannot treat the blood pressure without significant side-effects. Several of these tablets have a specific effect in preventing damage to your blood vessels from the effects of normal wear and tear and the diabetes itself.

Side-effects of tablets, if they do occur, depend on the type of tablet. One commonly used tablet sometimes causes an irritating cough. This is relieved when the tablet is changed. Another may produce slightly cold hands and feet and should be avoided in those with asthma. Details of side-effects should always be included on the information leaflet provided by your pharmacist but, remember, for legal reasons all possible side-effects are listed, however rare. Most people suffer no side-effects at all. If in doubt discuss this with your doctor before starting treatment.

Blood pressure does go up and down during the day. To achieve maximum benefit you need 24-hour control. Therefore, you should try to take the tablets at the times recommended.

Weight control and regular, and hopefully pleasurable, exercise help keep your blood pressure down. Smoking, however, has the reverse effect.

We recommend, therefore, that:

- Your blood pressure is checked at least annually
- You keep as good control of your weight as possible
- You avoid or stop smoking
- You try to take regular exercise
- If tablets are prescribed, you take them in the dose and at the time recommended.

The steps that you can take yourself may not only prevent the blood pressure rising but also, if it does need treating, help limit the number of tablets needed to keep it in the normal range. Side-effects of any tablets are therefore much less likely.

Blood cholesterol

A raised cholesterol level in the blood may aggravate a tendency to develop arterial disease. If the diabetes is poorly controlled the blood cholesterol is raised. In some individuals it is high, even when the blood glucose is normal. Over the age of 40 you should ask for a test (every five years). If it is persistently high, treatments are available which should help bring the level down to normal.

■ Damage to the feet

Foot problems are relatively common in your type of diabetes, but can usually be prevented with care. Therefore, this section is particularly important to you.

Long-term diabetes sometimes results in nerve damage (called neuritis or neuropathy). This mainly affects the feeling in the feet.

The feet normally undergo a lot of wear and tear, and any injuries are usually noticed because of discomfort. However, discomfort may not be felt because of neuropathy, and increasing damage to the feet may pass unnoticed. In addition, these injuries may be further aggravated by diminished circulation, which may lead to ulceration and infection. These can be very serious and result in prolonged periods off work, in bed, or in hospital, and sometimes require operations or even amputations.

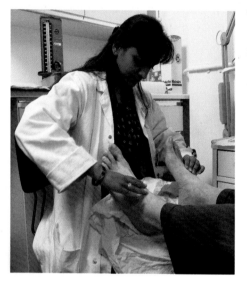

To a large extent these injuries can be avoided if proper care is taken of the feet. Foot care is of great importance, and you should read the following section carefully.

Prevention of foot problems

Scrupulous attention to care of the feet can prevent serious complications.

General measures for everyone

- Try to keep as good control of your diabetes as possible. This will keep the risk of any problems to a minimum.
- Avoid smoking. Nicotine is particularly harmful to the circulation of the lower legs and feet. The risk of severe changes is greatly increased if you continue to smoke.
- Be careful with your choice of footwear. Avoid shoes that rub, causing hard skin (callus) or blistering. Excess moisture may be a problem with sports shoes and lead to fungal infections.
- Wash your feet regularly and ensure that they are dried properly, especially between the toes.
- Learn how to cut your nails correctly.

Nail cutting

- When your toenails need cutting, do it after bathing, when the nails are soft and pliable. Do not cut them too short.
- Never cut the corners of your nails too far back at the sides, but allow the cut to follow the natural line of the end of the toe.
- Never use a sharp instrument to clean under your nails or in the nail grooves at the sides of the nails.
- If your toe nails are painful, or if you experience difficulty in cutting them, consult a state registered chiropodist/podiatrist.

Regular examination

- Make sure your feet are examined every year. This is the only way to find out whether greater care is necessary.

For older people and those with early nerve damage or circulatory problems

As you get older, and the longer you have diabetes, the chances of developing neuropathy and circulation problems increase a bit. You should be checked yearly for these and your doctor should tell you if there are any signs of this sort of damage. If so, follow the steps described below.

For those with definite neuropathy or circulatory problems and the elderly

These recommendations are essential. You should read them carefully. Scrupulous care can prevent serious problems.

Inspecting your feet

- Inspect your feet regularly – ideally, daily – and if you cannot do this yourself, ask a friend to do it for you. If you do it on your own a mirror on the floor or by the skirting board will help you. This inspection is important because you may not always be able to feel bruises or sores.
- Seek advice if you develop any cracks or breaks in the skin, any calluses or corns, or your feet are swollen or throbbing. Advice from a state registered chiropodist/podiatrist is freely available under the NHS.

Washing your feet

- Wash your feet daily in warm water. There is no advantage in soaking your feet – this makes the skin soggy at first and then dry, and more likely to become damaged.
- Use a mild type of soap.
- Rinse the skin well after washing. Dry your feet carefully, blotting between the toes with a soft towel.
- Dust with plain talc and wipe off any excess, so that it does not clog between the toes.
- Use moisturising cream after bathing, but do not apply cream between your toes as this area is usually moist enough.

Heat and cold

- Be careful to avoid baths that are too hot.
- Do not sit too close to heaters or fires.
- Before getting into bed, remove hot water bottles, unless they are fabric covered. Electric underblankets should be switched off or unplugged.
- If your feet get wet, dry them, and put on dry socks as soon as possible.
- Do not use hot fomentations or poultices.

Shoes

Shoes must fit properly and provide adequate support. In fact, careful fitting and choice of shoes is probably the most important measure you can take to prevent foot problems. Therefore:

- Wear well fitting shoes. They must be comfortable.
- Never accept shoes that have to be 'broken-in' before becoming comfortable.
- When buying new shoes, always try them on, and rely on the advice of a qualified shoe fitter. Shoes must always be the correct shape for your feet.
- Slippers do not provide adequate support and therefore should be worn only for short periods night and morning, and not throughout the day.
- Do not wear garters.
- Avoid walking barefoot.
- Daily rule – Feel inside your shoes and slippers before putting them on. This is important because you may not feel nails or stones under your feet as a result of loss of sensitivity in your feet.

Corns and calluses

- Do not cut corns and calluses yourself, or let a well meaning friend cut them for you.
- Do not use corn paints or corn plasters. They contain materials which can cause ulceration that might be difficult to heal.

First aid measures

- Minor injuries, such as cuts and abrasions, can be self-treated quite adequately, by gently cleaning the area with soap and water and covering it with a sterile dressing.
- If blisters occur, do not prick them. If they burst, dress them as for a minor cut.
- Never use strong medicaments, such as iodine, Dettol, Germaline or other powerful antiseptics.
- Never place adhesive strapping directly over a wound.
- If you are in the slightest doubt about how to deal with any wound, discoloration, corns, and especially ulcers, consult your doctor.

■ Painful neuropathy

Sometimes diabetic neuritis, or neuropathy as it is also known, causes pain. This is usually in the feet and legs and is particularly disagreeable. It builds up gradually. Typically, it causes a burning sensation, a feeling of pins and needles, with unpleasant discomfort on contact with clothes or bedclothes. It is usually worse in bed at night. Unpleasant though most of these symptoms are, they almost always disappear in time. It can, unfortunately, take many months for them to do so. Very good diabetes control is essential. Various treatments will help relieve the pain. Specialist advice is recommended.

Sexual function

Nerve damage can cause difficulty with erections (impotence). However, impotence is also common in those without diabetes. It is said that as many as 50 per cent of middle-aged men have quite long (but often temporary) periods of difficulty with erection. This is often for psychological reasons. Therefore, if you do have this problem, it may be difficult to be absolutely sure whether it is due to the nerve damage resulting from diabetes. Proper diagnosis is important and specialist advice should be sought from your doctor or from trained counsellors.

A variety of treatments are now available and these can be very successful. They include tablets and injections.

Viagra can be used providing you do not have heart problems and are receiving certain treatment for them. Alternative methods include injections which can be given into the penis. There are also a variety of devices which can help you obtain an erection.

Although it may seem embarrassing, do not hesitate to tell your doctor if you are concerned about this problem. Only in this way can a proper diagnosis be reached, with referral to an expert who should be able to help.

Other rare problems due to neuropathy

Very occasionally the part of the nervous system which controls the bowel, bladder and some other functions of the body may be damaged by diabetes.

With regard to the bowel, a rather unusual type of diarrhoea may develop. This tends to be explosive and particularly occurs at night. Fortunately it is usually quite intermittent.

Occasionally the nerves to the stomach may be affected. This causes delay of emptying and may cause nausea and sometimes vomiting.

The bladder may likewise be affected, with some difficulty in emptying the bladder when you pass urine.

Finally, as opposed to high blood pressure, the pressure may fall when you stand up. This is usually manifested by a slight dizziness.

It should be stressed that these are very unusual complications and they only occur after many years of diabetes. Special treatments are now available which help relieve these problems. Therefore if you feel you have symptoms which concern you, do tell your doctor about them.

◼ Damage to the eyes

Two parts of the eye are affected by diabetes.

1. The lens: Opacities in the lens (cataracts) are common in elderly people and sometimes cause deterioration of vision. Cataracts are more common in older people with diabetes.
2. The retina: This is the sensitive part of the back of the eye. The damage that can be caused by diabetes is called diabetic retinopathy. This takes several years to develop. Usually abnormalities are minor and cause no loss of vision. In a minority of people, however, this retinopathy can progress and vision can deteriorate. Without early treatment the affected eye may become blind, usually from bleeding (haemorrhage) within the eye.

Prevention and treatment of eye damage

Cataracts can interfere with vision. However, in the early stages they may cause no problems. They will, if present, be detected at your routine yearly eye examination. If this is the case do not be too alarmed. It may be several years before they interfere with vision. When this happens they can be treated by a simple and straightforward operation. A new artificial lens will almost always restore sight to normal.

Damage to the retina fortunately can now be treated. Blindness should not occur. Treatment is by laser, a process which involves aiming a fine beam

of very bright light at the abnormal blood vessel. It is simple to perform and is usually successful. But it does have to be undertaken before sight has deteriorated too seriously. Therefore, it is essential that you should have your eyes tested and the back of your eyes examined regularly – ideally annually. This can be done by an optician, by doctors in the diabetes clinic or by an eye specialist.

Remember, some blurring of vision may occur in the first few weeks of treatment. This is usually of no consequence and nearly always resolves within a week or two, so do not get your glasses changed. However, if you should notice a sudden loss of vision in either eye, you must report to your doctor immediately.

Contact lenses

People with diabetes should be aware that they have a higher risk of developing irritation of the eye from contact lens usage than those without diabetes. A meticulous cleaning routine and careful technique for lens handling are important. You should make sure that you have been shown how to do this and you should have your technique checked from time to time. If you are using daily-wear soft lenses, these should be exchanged every six months.

Extended-wear soft lenses should not generally be prescribed for those with diabetes, as damage to the cornea is more common with this type. If your eyes become red or irritated, you should immediately stop using contact lenses and seek advice.

◼ Damage to the kidneys

Damage to the kidneys (usually called nephropathy) occurs less frequently than eye damage. The damage to the kidneys must have been present for many years before function begins to deteriorate. Even then a few more years usually elapse before the situation becomes serious. Unfortunately kidney disease does not give rise to symptoms until it is quite advanced. Early detection by means of regular checks from your doctor is very important. There is now a test that can be performed on your urine which gives an indication of early damage. These tests become positive at a stage when the deterioration can be delayed. In the case of severe kidney damage the same treatment given to those with other causes can be provided for those with diabetes.

◼ Diabetes and other illnesses

The effect of illness on diabetes

In the section on treatment (see page 58) it was indicated that under certain circumstances your diabetes may go temporarily out of control. Although loss of control for a few days is of no real significance, if you should develop symptoms of thirst and dryness of the mouth or pass large quantities of urine, you should consult your doctor.

Diabetes and the treatment of other illnesses

Diabetes is no bar to the treatment – including operations – of any other disorder or illness. Your diabetes may not be so easily controlled during any illness or after an operation. Adjustment of your diabetes treatment may be necessary.

Certain drugs may cause a rise in blood glucose (eg steroids and water tablets). Adjustment of their doses or your diabetes treatment may be necessary.

Dentistry

Routine dental treatment can be carried out by your dentist in the normal way. If, however, you are taking insulin special precautions may be needed and you should consult your doctor.

Associated illnesses

Very occasionally, diabetes may be associated with another illness, or it may actually be part of another illness. Sometimes diabetes apparently develops as a result of the treatment given for other illnesses. Disorders of the liver and pancreas, excess iron stores in the body, and hormonal problems involving the thyroid and adrenal glands are quite often associated with diabetes. Generally, such problems will be identified when you first see your doctor. Treatment will be prescribed in parallel with the treatment for your diabetes.

Vaccination

With diabetes you can be vaccinated in exactly the same way as those without diabetes. Sometimes vaccinations cause a mild fever a day or two later. This may cause your blood glucose level to rise. Don't be alarmed by this, these effects pass in 24–48 hours.

There are certain vaccinations which are recommended for those with diabetes. They are vaccinations against flu and pneumonia. For younger people who are fit and well they are not really necessary. However, they do provide some protection for older people, especially those who have other problems such as heart or lung disorders.

OUTPATIENT APPOINTMENTS

Name _____

Address _____

_____

Date	Time	Consultant	Clinic

Bring this card with you to the hospital

Diabetes control whilst in hospital

When you are in hospital you may be confined to bed and will not be taking any exercise. You may be anxious, and your diet will most probably be different. Together these factors undoubtedly cause your blood tests to rise. Consequently, your diabetes treatment will need to be increased. Tablets may be introduced for the first time, or their dose increased. Sometimes insulin will be recommended, almost always on a temporary basis. You should realise that the cause of these changes in your diabetes control is the result of prevailing circumstances, and not a failure on the part of yourself or of the hospital staff.

You may wish to continue your own tests and adjust your own diabetes treatment when in hospital. This is now permissible in most circumstances. Ask the ward staff if you wish to do so.

■ Clinic attendance

The organisation of clinics

Your local diabetes clinic plays an important role in helping you control your diabetes and detecting and treating any complications. The organisation of these clinics varies in different areas of the country. In some cases it is at the local hospital and is under the direction of a hospital consultant. Many units have set up special diabetes centres with expertly trained doctors, nurses, dietitians and chiropodists/podiatrists. In many districts clinics have been established in specially trained general practices, or cooperative schemes have been developed between hospital specialists and family doctors. Evening clinics may be held to enable you to attend after work.

■ Regular medical review

In the period after your diabetes has been diagnosed, your doctor may wish to see you every few weeks, until he or she is sure that the treatment is effective. However, when your blood glucose has been brought under control, you may only need to attend perhaps every few months.

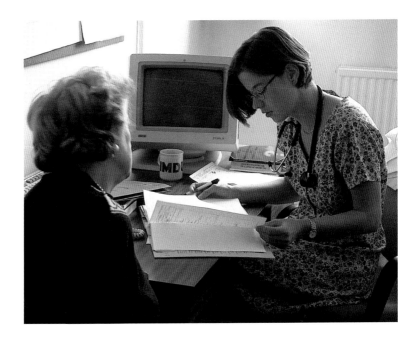

With your urine or blood test records you will be able to keep a routine check on the effectiveness of your treatment. None the less, from time to time it is essential that you visit your doctor or clinic so that your treatment can be monitored, and any specific problems you may have can be dealt with.

- Your doctor will be concerned to know that your glucose control is satisfactory. If the record of your tests shows erratic or high glucose levels, he or she will decide whether additional treatment is necessary.
- You should have the long-term averaging test (Haemoglobin A_{1c} or fructosamine). This gives an indication of your overall average blood glucose control (see page 52).
- Your doctor will want to ensure that you understand and are happy with the advice you have been given. This is the time for you to ask questions!
- From time to time, you do have to be checked to see whether any long-term complications have developed. It is important that these should be detected before you notice anything wrong, so that early treatment can be commenced.
- Finally, such visits provide you with an opportunity to discuss problems with, for example, your dietitian. You should also report any new symptoms, such as difficulty with vision or problems with your feet.

Once your diabetes is reasonably controlled you should:

1. See a specialist and/or practice nurse, doctor, dietitian and chiropodist at regular intervals – annually, or more often if necessary. These meetings should give time for discussion as well as for assessing your control.
2. Be able to contact any member of the healthcare team for specialist advice when you need it.
3. Have more education sessions as you are ready for them.
4. Have a formal medical review at least once a year by a doctor experienced in diabetes. This review should include the following.

   - Your weight should be recorded.
   - Your urine should be tested for protein.
   - Your blood should be tested to measure long-term control.
   - You should discuss control, including your home monitoring results.
   - Your blood pressure should be checked.
   - Your vision should be checked, and the backs of your eyes examined. To do this your pupils have to be dilated. This requires some drops being put into your eyes. This is in no way harmful. They may sting a bit for a minute or so. If necessary you should be referred to an ophthalmologist.

However, you need to be warned that there may be some blurring of vision for a while after this. You are advised, therefore, not to drive on this occasion, or if you do you must be careful. It can be particularly uncomfortable if it is a very bright day, and you would be advised to use some dark glasses. The blurring wears off, usually within quite a short time, and no long-term effects occur.

   - Your legs and feet should be examined to check your circulation and nerve supply. If necessary you should be referred to a chiropodist/podiatrist.
   - Your injection sites should be examined if you are on insulin.
   - You should have the opportunity to discuss how you are coping at home and at work.
   - Beyond the age of 40 it is wise to have your cholesterol checked. If the result is normal, this test only needs to be repeated every five years.

The control of your diabetes is important, and so are the detection and treatment of any complications. Make sure you are getting the medical care and education you need to ensure you stay healthy. If you are not feeling well, your treatment appears not to be working, or if you develop any unusual symptoms such as worsening eyesight, or abnormal tingling in the hands or feet, report this to your doctor at once – DO NOT WAIT FOR YOUR NEXT APPOINTMENT.

■ Summary

It must be stressed that most of the problems of long-term diabetes can normally be avoided, or the risks greatly reduced.

Remember:

- Good control of diabetes usually prevents the development of these complications. Therefore, advice from regular clinic attendance is very important.
- Smoking accelerates arterial disease (affecting the heart and feet), and may also have a bad effect on your eyes and kidneys.
- Try to control your weight.
- Keep a regular eye on your own tests.

8 Diabetes and Your Daily Life

This chapter answers some of the most frequently asked questions about the influence of diabetes on your everyday activities. It discusses topics such as the financial implications of diabetes, and the additional steps you may need to take in order to remain fit and active.

Type 2 diabetes is, in the majority of cases, easily controlled by diet, or by diet and tablets, and should therefore make very little difference to your daily life. Undoubtedly, the greatest change will be the need to modify and regulate your diet, but other day-to-day activities should need to be altered very little.

■ Employment

Diabetes and its influence on your work

For the vast majority of people with Type 2 diabetes, their condition has no effect on their work. Consequently, your ability to function well should be as good as before you developed diabetes, perhaps even better. There are, however, certain careers in which having diabetes can prove a hindrance.

- If your work involves driving a passenger-carrying vehicle, and you have to take insulin for the treatment of your diabetes, then certain restrictions may be imposed.
- Because of statutory regulations, you will not be allowed to fly aeroplanes.
- In some occupations, employers impose rather strict health regulations. For example, you cannot be accepted for entry into the armed services, although if you are an established member you should be able to continue without difficulty.
- If you have a potentially highly dangerous job, eg deep-sea diving, steeplejacking, or any job for which very high standards of fitness are required, you will probably have to change your occupation.

Diabetes and your employer

Unless you work in one of the occupations mentioned above, your employer need have no fears about your ability to continue employment or commence a new job. Unfortunately, some employers do not know very much about diabetes and are therefore often reluctant to employ anybody with diabetes, in the mistaken belief that they might prove to be an unreliable employee. Therefore, you should stress to your employer that with uncomplicated diabetes you are as capable of performing your job as a person without diabetes, and without risk to yourself or others. Shift work should pose no problems and, unlike those with insulin treated diabetes, you do not require specific breaks for snacks or additional meals.

Occasionally, employers will not employ people with diabetes, because of their fear of future problems. In particular, they may be apprehensive that late complications may develop and render an employee incapable of full-time work.

If you experience difficulty in convincing your employer that you are fit to take up a new job, or to continue in your existing one, enlist the help of your family doctor or your hospital doctor and, if necessary, Diabetes UK. You may have rights under the Disability Discrimination Act.

■ Financial implications of having diabetes

Insurance

Having diabetes should not give rise to any serious financial problems. You may experience some increased expenditure, however, in the field of life insurance. In all matters relating to insurance, it is essential to be completely frank with brokers or insurers. Concealment of any important medical facts may invalidate the insurance offered, with potentially serious financial and legal consequences. There is no need, however, to inform your insurance company of your diabetes for any life policies taken out before your diagnosis.

Motor insurance

If you hold a motor insurance policy, you must notify your insurance company or insurance broker immediately that you develop diabetes, although many companies no longer record their information. Failure to do so may cause liability to be denied in the event of a claim. Most insurance companies will continue to offer cover to clients who develop diabetes. Some companies may require a medical certificate from your doctor. Attempts to impose an additional premium because of the diabetes should be resisted.

If you encounter difficulties, details of the Diabetes UK's Insurance Services may be obtained from Diabetes UK.

Life insurance

Because of the possibility of long-term complications developing, it is normal for some loading to be placed on life and health insurance policies. If your diabetes is perfectly controlled and you have no complications, this loading should be small, but may be 5–10 per cent on whole life policies. Loading for term assurance, eg mortgage protection or endowment policies, will be higher, but will normally be less than for those who are treated with insulin. If you experience any problems, you should seek help from Diabetes UK. Diabetes UK Insurance Services also offer life cover.

Sickness, accident and holiday insurance

It is essential that you declare your diabetes when taking out life or health insurance. Those with diabetes seeking personal sickness and accident insurance are likely to have to pay higher than normal premiums.

Those taking out insurance in connection with travel and holidays abroad must pay particular attention to the exclusion clauses. They normally exclude all pre-existing illnesses, ie those present before you travel. However, special cover for people with diabetes can usually be arranged, and Diabetes UK can give advice on this matter. Do not forget that failing to declare your diabetes when taking out travel insurance could nullify the policy.

Pensions and superannuation

Your pension rights should be unaffected by your diabetes. If you enter into a new scheme, it is essential that you declare your diabetes.

Other financial considerations

■ Prescription charges in the UK are waived for people with diabetes treated with tablets and insulin, but not if the diabetes is treated by diet alone. FP92M will be signed by you so that you may obtain an exemption certificate. This applies to all prescriptions, whether related to your diabetes or not.

- Everybody with diabetes is entitled to free eye tests.
- Some people may find that they have to spend more money on buying a healthy diet, and on such items as suitable footwear. If you are dependent on Social Security for your income, it may be worthwhile contacting your local Citizens Advice Bureau or Welfare Rights Service to make sure that you are getting your full entitlement.
- Those who develop late complications, especially with their eyes, may be eligible for additional benefits.

■ Driving

Points to remember

- Tell your insurance company that you have diabetes.

- If your diabetes is treated with tablets or insulin you must tell the licensing authorities (Drivers Medical Branch, DVLA, Swansea SA99 1TU) that you have diabetes.

Applying for a driving licence

When you apply for a driving licence you have to answer a question on whether you have diabetes.

To this question you should answer 'Yes', whether you have diabetes treated with insulin, or diet and tablets, or diet alone. In the space provided for details, you should state that you have diabetes, adding that your diabetes is controlled by diet, diet and tablets, or insulin, as appropriate. If your diabetes is treated with diet alone or diet and tablets, no further action will be taken and your 'till 70' licence will remain valid.

However you must notify the DVLA immediately if the treatment of your diabetes is changed or if you develop any complications.

If you are taking insulin, after you have completed and returned your application form, you will be sent another form, asking for further information. This will include the name and address of your doctor or hospital clinic, as well as your consent for the Driver and Vehicle Licensing Authority to approach your doctor for a detailed report on your diabetes. This complication of procedure does not mean that you will be refused a driving licence. The licence will normally be issued without delay for three years and renewals will be made free of charge.

If your diabetes was diagnosed only recently, and you are started on insulin and you already hold a 'life' licence, this will be revoked and replaced with a 'period' licence. This is renewable every three years. Renewals can take several weeks, but should your licence pass its expiry date, you can continue to drive providing you have made application for a renewal. Heavy goods vehicle (Group 2) licences and passenger-carrying vehicle licences are not prohibited to those with uncomplicated diabetes who do not take insulin. Some restrictions will be imposed if you have problems with your eyesight or other significant disabilities.

If, however, you have to start insulin treatment and you drive heavy goods vehicles, Group 2 (greater than 3.5 tonnes – but see page 111), or minibuses or hold a passenger vehicle licence you will be subject to yearly review by a specialist. With regard to ordinary driving licences, these will not be revoked should you have to start insulin. This means you can continue to drive cars, motorcycles, vans and lorries up to 3.5 tonnes and minibuses for nine people or less. More care, however, is required – see page 68.

Taking care

If you have diabetes controlled by diet alone, and have normal eyesight (with glasses if necessary), there are no special precautions which you need to take.

If, however, you take tablets:

- You must ensure that you have your meals regularly.
- You should not drive if you are already late for a meal. If you have any problems obtaining a driving licence, you should contact Diabetes UK.

■ Exercise and sport

As described in Chapter 3 about your treatment, the more exercise you can take the better it is for your diabetes. Certainly no restrictions are needed in uncomplicated diabetes.

Exercise is an important aspect of the overall programme to control your diabetes. It not only lowers your blood glucose, it makes the action of insulin on your fat and muscle cells more efficient. Therefore exercise is very beneficial and is actively encouraged. There is no reason why you should not be able to continue heavy manual work, or continue to enjoy any of the sports you played before your diabetes was diagnosed. There are leading tennis and badminton players, golfers, swimmers, cricketers, athletes and professional footballers who have diabetes.

Unlike a person with Type 1 diabetes, there is usually no need for you to adjust your diet before strenuous exercise. If you are taking tablets, however, your blood glucose may fall lower than usual during exercise. This can be readily put right by an extra snack of carbohydrate-containing food.

If you are a more sedentary type of person, not given to playing sport, you should, if possible, take routine, moderate exercise. Regular walking, for example, is better than short bursts of very strenuous exercise, and it can do much to preserve and even improve the circulation. Although a great deal of such mild exercise may be needed to reduce weight, it can make a contribution towards this goal. Keeping fit is an essential aspect of maintaining good diabetes control.

Keeping fit is an essential aspect of maintaining good diabetes control

■ Retirement

All retired people have to adjust to stopping the normal routine of going to work, and to the fact that they are no longer associating with colleagues and workmates. Loss of such contacts and interests may lead to bouts of depression, particularly in those who have never developed hobbies or interests outside their work. However, as long as you are otherwise fit, retirement should cause no greater problems for you than for anybody else.

If you are retired, it is essential that you should not allow your diabetes to stop you from developing new interests, or from making an active contribution to the community. For example, you could undertake voluntary work for Diabetes UK or other charitable organisations.

Do not forget to take advantage of the various benefits available to you as a retired person. Reduced fares on public transport and reduced entrance fees to certain places of entertainment, for example, could provide you with many opportunities not previously enjoyed.

Don't let your diabetes stop
you from enjoying a full
and active retirement

Maintaining careful control of your diabetes, and taking whatever exercise is possible, are the best ways to ensure that you remain healthy into old age.

Remember to ask your doctor or dietitian about adjustments to your diet if your activity level increases or decreases.

■ Travel and holidays

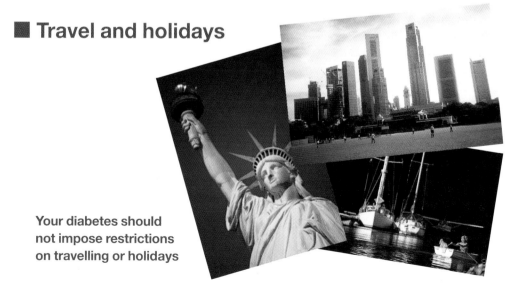

Your diabetes should
not impose restrictions
on travelling or holidays

It is wise, however, to take certain essential precautions, bearing in mind that even people without diabetes frequently suffer unforeseen circumstances away from home.

Illness

Mild gastroenteritis is an ailment commonly suffered while travelling abroad, and could cause your diabetes to go temporarily out of control.

Whenever you feel unwell whilst travelling, test your urine or blood glucose. If the results show a high glucose reading, and you feel very dry and thirsty, consult a doctor. Most of the illnesses you are likely to experience while away from home will be mild and of short duration. All you may notice are positive urine tests or high blood tests for a day or so, which then return to normal.

These are the most important points to remember when travelling at home or abroad:

- Take your diabetes testing equipment with you.
- If you take tablets or insulin, carry more than you are likely to require. This is particularly important when travelling abroad, in case your return should be delayed.
- When travelling overseas, always take out health insurance.
- Always carry a card indicating that you have diabetes – this is essential if you take tablets or insulin.

Insulin user's identity card

Diabetes UK

AFFIX PHOTO HERE

- If I am found ill, please give me some form of sugar such as chocolate, sweets, fizzy...
- If I fail to re~~ plea~~ glucose.

I have diabetes

Name

Address

Telephone

In an emergency please contact

Always carry some form of identification

Foreign food

Eating different food, cooked in an unfamiliar way, may cause some problems, especially when eating out. Usually, though, you will find little difficulty in recognising food similar to that of your normal diet. Alternative starchy carbohydrate staple foods will be available, eg couscous, local breads, rice, etc.

An occasional deviation from your normal diet will do no harm, and may merely cause an isolated positive urine test or high blood test. If, however, you are overweight and have been on a diet, do not spoil all your previous good work.

Air travel

You are not subject to any special restrictions, and you need take no special precautions. If you take tablets for your diabetes and are going on long-distance flights, don't worry too much about the exact timing. Just try to space them at least 10 hours apart. If you miss one dose you will come to no harm. If you can take insulin, you should discuss this with your diabetes team.

Many airlines offer special 'diabetic' meals. However, these often have very little carbohydrate. It is usually better to choose the normal meal, especially as the portions tend to be small.

Vaccinations

Diabetes does not impose any restrictions on the vaccinations you may need if travelling abroad. However, immunisation against certain illnesses may be followed by a day or so of feeling mildly unwell, together with a temporary rise in your blood glucose. This should cause you no concern.

Travel guides

Travel guides for many of the popular tourist destinations are available from Diabetes UK. Contact Diabetes UK for further information.

■ Contraception, pregnancy and parenthood

Contraception

Because Type 2 diabetes usually occurs in women who are middle-aged, contraception may not be a matter of concern. If, however, you are of an appropriate age, then you should seek advice on contraception from your doctor or family planning clinic. Although the risk to a woman's health from the normal contraceptive pill is very low, in your case your diabetes may increase this risk slightly. The contraceptive pill may also lead to a rise in blood glucose, in which case other forms of contraception may be advisable.

Pregnancy

Diabetes should not prevent you from getting married and having a family

If you are a woman of child-bearing age and you intend having a child, there are several very important things you should do:

1. You must ensure that your diabetes is well controlled when you are planning the pregnancy.
2. It is absolutely essential that, once you know you are pregnant, you achieve perfect control and maintain it throughout pregnancy. The reason for this is that your growing baby, even though it will not have diabetes, will be subject to your insulin and blood glucose levels.
3. If you take diabetes tablets these should be stopped as soon as you know you are pregnant. You should consult a specialist in diabetes, ideally before you conceive.

4. All women are now advised to start taking folic acid for one month before conception, if possible.

Therefore, if you are planning a pregnancy, and certainly as soon as you become pregnant, you must contact your doctor and/or hospital clinic. Also, in order to make sure that your pregnancy continues without problems, you must attend your diabetes clinic regularly.

You may find that you require additional treatment during pregnancy, or even a period in hospital. Such special measures can usually be stopped as soon as the baby has been delivered. With care from yourself and your doctor, a successful outcome is the rule.

Diabetes and heredity

The question asked by most parents is: 'What are the chances of my child having diabetes?' There is no easy answer to this question, because the way in which diabetes is inherited is a complex process, which is not yet fully understood. In Type 2 diabetes it does appear that inheritance plays a more significant role than in Type 1 diabetes. It must be stressed that it is most unlikely that any of your children will develop diabetes during childhood, as most inherited diabetes develops only later in life.

Many people who inherit the tendency to develop diabetes never actually do so. This is because other factors, including damage to the pancreas, emotional factors, obesity, and in some instances even viral infections, are necessary for the development of diabetes.

■ The effect on your family

When you are first told that you have diabetes, a chronic lifelong condition, you may well feel confused and upset. This is a very normal reaction, and you may find that your family feel equally worried by the diagnosis. Talking about these feelings with each other, with the health professionals involved in your diabetes care, and with other people with diabetes and their families can help.

With time, the majority of people come to terms with their diabetes, as they learn more about it. This learning about diabetes is recognised as a very important part of the treatment. Equally important is keeping your family up to date with this information. Most clinics will encourage you to bring someone with you for educational sessions. The people around you will be more able to give you the help and support you need to live with your diabetes, if they have the same information as you.

If the members of your family want to understand more about diabetes, the local group of Diabetes UK can also be very helpful, and membership is open to the whole family.

■ Who is available to help?

With diet and tablets you should be able to control your diabetes. From time to time, however, you may develop problems about which you need specialist advice. On such occasions you may refer to a variety of individuals, including your doctor, nurses, dietitians, chiropodists, the Social Services and, of course, your local hospital clinic.

In the next chapter we also describe the help available to you from Diabetes UK.

■ Some final comments on diabetes and your everyday life

- ■ With relatively straightforward modifications to your daily life, effective control of your blood glucose level is possible.
- ■ Make the necessary changes to your diet and try to stick to them.
- ■ Lose some weight if you need to and keep it off!
- ■ If you need to take tablets, take them regularly.
- ■ Take reasonable care of your general health, and your feet in particular.
- ■ Attend your clinic for regular check-ups.

The late Dr R D Lawrence, physician and co-founder of the British Diabetic Association (now Diabetes UK), wrote in his famous book *The Diabetic Life*:

> There is no reason why a diabetic should not, if he can be taught to do so, lead a long and normal life. True, the diabetic life demands self-control from all its subjects, but it gives in return a full and active existence, with no real privations.

9 Diabetes UK

Being diagnosed with diabetes can leave you feeling very confused and isolated. If you have lots of unanswered questions about your diabetes, need advice on how diabetes might affect your home life or your work, or want to be put in touch with other people with diabetes, contact Diabetes UK. The organisation is here to work with you to improve the level of diabetes care available. It is a medical self-help charity that has both lay and professional members, and has been working with people with diabetes for over 60 years. This chapter describes Diabetes UK's work and invites you to support them.

■ Diabetes UK's history

Diabetes UK (the new name for the British Diabetic Association) was founded in 1934 by R D Lawrence, a diabetologist who had diabetes himself, and H G Wells, the author of books such as *The Time Machine* and *War of the Worlds*. The organisation's aims remain the same as they were in the 1930s: to help and care for people with diabetes and those close to them, to represent and campaign for their interests, and to fund research into diabetes. But advances in medical and information technology since the charity was founded mean that today Diabetes UK can pursue these goals in ways that even H G Wells could never have foreseen.

■ Providing care and advice

Diabetes UK Careline

To help you understand and manage your diabetes Diabetes UK runs a careline. Diabetes UK Careline is a confidential service which offers

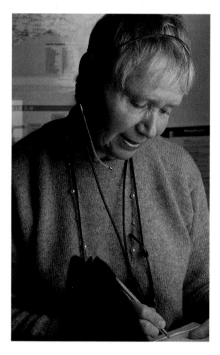

information and support on diabetes by telephone, letter, fax or email. Diabetes UK Careline staff cannot comment on your individual medical situation – your doctor or specialist nurse is in the best position to do this – but they can talk over any difficulties you may be having and send you information on a wide range of diabetes-related subjects.

Diabetes UK Careline staff are trained in diabetes and also have counselling experience. You may wish to talk in confidence about a difficult or distressing situation; you do not have to give your name or address to receive help.

Diabetes UK Careline deals with calls and letters on a wide range of subjects related to diabetes, including hypoglycaemia, complications, employment, driving, schools, holidays, blood glucose testing and many, many more. Sometimes the phone lines are very busy so you may not always get through the first time you try.

Diabetes UK Careline's telephone number is 020 7636 6112, Textphone (for hard of hearing and deaf) 020 7462 2757. The lines are open Monday to Friday, 9 am–5 pm. Careline can also be contacted by fax: on 020 7462 2732 and by email: careline@diabetes.org.uk.

Care Developments

The Care Developments team support Diabetes UK Careline staff and provides the organisation with nursing and diabetes expertise.

The team's role is to ensure that Diabetes UK keeps up to date with developments in diabetes and produces information sheets and leaflets for people with diabetes on all aspects of living with the condition.

Care Developments also provide information through *Balance*, Diabetes UK's bimonthly magazine, and through our website, as well as responding to individual enquiries.

Care Interventions

The Care Interventions team works to identify and develop activity and information for people with diabetes at key points in their lives.

The Youth and Family Events section runs educational holidays and family weekend events for families with a child with diabetes. These annual events offer families an opportunity to meet others and discuss and address ways forward to improve their understanding and management of the condition.

In addition, the Project Development section is continually developing new activities to support people with diabetes at and around the time of diagnosis.

■ Sharing experiences

Adjusting to the knowledge that you or a member of your family has diabetes takes time and it is often helpful to meet other people who live with diabetes and have been through a similar situation. They can offer understanding, help and support at an important time. A good way of finding this help is to join a local Diabetes UK voluntary group. There are over 400 across Britain and Northern Ireland, all run voluntarily by people living with diabetes. There are also some specialist groups – for parents and young people with diabetes, South Asian support groups and a group for the visually impaired.

If you would like more information about the groups network, contact Diabetes UK's Voluntary Groups Section. All voluntary groups welcome new members.

Every year, Diabetes UK also organises around 10 *Living with Diabetes* days, which take place on various Saturdays throughout the UK. These take the form of one-day conferences and exhibitions on diabetes, giving you an introduction to life with the condition, how healthcare professionals can help you, and the latest in diabetes research. The conference is accompanied by an exhibition presented by companies from the pharmaceutical industry who will be promoting their services and products.

■ Spreading the word

Communications are an essential part of Diabetes UK's work. The organisation is uniquely placed to draw together information related to diabetes from the points of view of people with diabetes, carers, healthcare professionals and researchers. As a result, Diabetes UK publishes information which can inform and represent all of these groups, as well as improve the general public's understanding of diabetes.

Leaflets and magazines

It is often useful to have your queries backed up with written information, which you can digest later and refer back to. Diabetes UK is the foremost source of leaflets, magazines and books on diabetes – in fact, it has many titles to help you understand more about your condition. Many of the leaflets are free of charge, a number of our publications are available in Welsh and the major Asian languages, and some are available on tape.

In addition to leaflets on single subjects such as *Eating Well*, *Diabetes and Insurance*, and *Treating your Diabetes with Tablets*, Diabetes UK also publishes *Balance*, a bimonthly magazine for Diabetes UK members. *Balance* is filled with news, interviews, research updates, recipes and diet information, showing you how you can fit diabetes into an active lifestyle. It is also available on tape and can be bought at larger branches of W H Smith and newsagents. Diabetes UK also publishes a series called *Diabetes for Beginners*, aimed at helping newly diagnosed people.

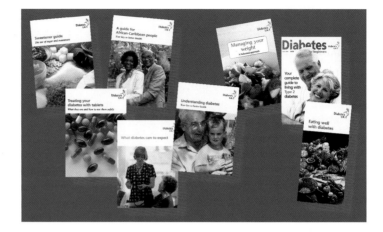

The website

The Internet is a great way both of communicating with other people and of providing information to help you learn more about diabetes. Diabetes UK relaunched its website in June 2000. The site has all the latest news and up to date information on diabetes. It covers all areas of diabetes, from *What is diabetes?* And *Managing diabetes*, through to local support and getting involved with Diabetes UK. The online information centre is a particularly useful resource, containing all of Diabetes UK's free publications. There is also a section devoted to research and an area for healthcare professionals. You can find Diabetes UK at http://www.diabetes.org.uk.

Networks for healthcare professionals

Professional Conferences

Another important function of Diabetes UK is to spread the news about the latest research and up-to-date guidelines on good diabetes care among the healthcare professionals, eg GPs, nurses, chiropodists and dietitians, who are involved in diabetes care. A number of publications are available to this end, including professional reports setting out recommendations for diabetes care and *Diabetes Update*, a quarterly newsletter for all members of the diabetes care team. There are Medical and Scientific Conferences, held twice a year, which now attract up to 1000 participants. These allow health-care professionals and scientists to network and give them the opportunity to hear lectures on the latest diabetes research and the various scientific and clinical aspects of the condition.

Poster campaigns

Finally, through its poster campaigns the Diabetes UK sets out to raise public awareness and funds, and to reach people who may have diabetes but haven't yet been diagnosed. This last is a particularly urgent task given that in the UK alone an estimated one million people are thought to have undetected Type 2 non insulin dependent diabetes. The longer their diabetes goes undetected, the greater their risk of developing complications.

■ Fighting discrimination

Event days and poster campaigns are an important means of raising public awareness of diabetes, and in this way, they are also a key weapon in the fight against discrimination: the more people know about diabetes, the less likely they are to discriminate against people with diabetes. Nevertheless, a good deal of progress still needs to be made in this area, and Diabetes UK is active in opposing discrimination against people with diabetes.

Employment

One major field of discrimination is the job market. Often this sort of discrimination is the result of ignorant outdated ideas about what people with diabetes can and can't do, and may be appealed against under the Disability Discrimination Act. Diabetes UK's Diabetes Care Services can provide you with some of the information you may need to do this.

In some occupations, however, job applicants may come up against an official 'blanket' ban on people with diabetes. Diabetes UK believes that each person with diabetes should be treated as a case in their own right, and has made this argument very successfully in a number of areas of work. It also gives guidance to individuals who find it hard to challenge discrimination. For example, it was decided that firefighters who are diagnosed in service with Type 1 diabetes will no longer be dismissed immediately. Decisions will now be made on a case-by-case basis. Our campaigning work also led to a government review of regulations that originally barred insulin-users from driving vehicles above 3.5 tonnes at work.

Insurance

Another area where people with diabetes have been discriminated against in the past is insurance. Discrimination may come in the form of increased premiums, restricted terms or even cancellation of policies. Diabetes UK Careline used to receive thousands of calls each year from people having problems finding or keeping their driving insurance cover. This situation has been radically improved by the Disability Discrimination Act, but some companies do still charge higher premiums. Revealing that you have diabetes may be problematic, but keeping it a secret from your insurers is even worse. Failure to disclose material facts can invalidate your insurance cover in the event of a claim.

Travel insurance can still be problematic; many travel insurance policies do not include pre-existing medical conditions such as diabetes, so it is important to check carefully before arranging your holiday. As with other policies, the consequences of not mentioning your diabetes may be disastrous, leaving you liable to enormous medical bills.

As far as life assurance policies are concerned, if you already hold a policy when you are diagnosed, you don't need to declare your diabetes. But if you are applying for a new policy you must declare it and expect some loading on your policy.

Faced with the general lack of understanding within the insurance market, Diabetes UK has negotiated its own exclusive schemes to provide policies suited to the needs of people with diabetes and those living with them. Diabetes UK Services offer competitively priced motor and travel insurance, as well as life and home insurance, and other investment products.

■ Leading the way to better care

Through the campaigning activities of Diabetes UK members, considerable improvements in care have been achieved both in hospital clinics and general practice. Over recent years, Diabetes UK has also secured disposable insulin syringes, needles and blood glucose testing strips on NHS prescription. In March 2000, needles and reusable insulin pens also became free to people with diabetes.

Diabetes UK is working closely with the Department of Health on a Diabetes National Service framework, which aims to ensure high standards of care consistently across England. Similar cooperation with government is taking place in Scotland, Wales and Northern Ireland.

Diabetes UK is actively encouraging the development of Local Diabetes Services Advisory Groups (LDSAGs) in local health authorities around the country.

Local Diabetes Services Advisory Groups

An LDSAG is a group of people whose purpose is to be involved in the formation of a local strategy for diabetes services, to advise on and monitor its effects and to recommend the improvements required to provide a service which meets local needs and wishes and national standards. The role and responsibilities of LDSAGs include:

- ■ Developing a local strategy for diabetes care and prevention, with specific objectives and targets.
- ■ Advising on the development of service specification to meet those needs.
- ■ Developing systems to facilitate the achievement of the targets and user satisfaction.
- ■ Monitoring and auditing the quality of the service against the targets and standards set.
- ■ Developing a local information system to assist in this process and identify shortfalls.

Membership includes: representatives of the specialist team and the primary healthcare team, people with diabetes and their carers, commissioners of diabetes services, consultants in public health medicine, managers of provider services, representatives of Diabetes UK voluntary groups and community health centres.

Other members may come from relevant medical specialities, social services, education, health promotion, other voluntary organisations and other relevant local groups or individuals.

Professional membership

Through its professional membership there is close communication between the professionals and Diabetes UK so that its advice and policies are based on and have the support of its professional members. Nearly all doctors specialising in diabetes and specialist nurses, many dietitians and large numbers of general practitioners are members. Primary Care Diabetes UK, one of the professional membership sections, was established to improve co-ordination of care in general practice. The organisation is committed to encouraging high-quality and culturally sensitive primary care for people with diabetes.

The St Vincent Declaration

A significant guide to Diabetes UK's work is the *St Vincent Declaration*, a document compiled in 1989 by diabetes organisations, healthcare professionals and people with diabetes. This sets out targets for reducing the complications of diabetes throughout Europe by improving the way diabetes care is provided.

■ Searching for a cure

Diabetes research is very exciting at the moment, with a number of areas of research at critical stages of development. Diabetes UK is very active in supporting this research. There are usually around 150 Diabetes UK-funded research projects going on throughout the UK, investigating the causes, treatment and prevention of diabetes. Scientists are also looking at hypos, how complications can be prevented, better ways of screening and new targets for treatment design. There are even studies underway looking at some of the psychological aspects of diabetes and what types of diabetes education are most effective.

Diabetes UK is one of the largest funders of diabetes research in the UK. The organisation believes in funding only the highest quality research that promises to make the maximum impact on diabetes. Diabetes UK has two committees: the Research Committee and the Diabetes Development Committee, which between them meet five times each year to decide exactly how money will be spent.

The money for research comes mainly from voluntary sources in the form of donations and legacies. People can ask for their donation to be set aside specifically for our Research Fund or they can support research on a regular basis by joining Diabetes UK Research Focus. Please call our Customer Services on 020 7462 2791 for further information.

■ How you can help

Diabetes UK relies upon its supporters – people with diabetes, their families and friends, and healthcare professionals working in the field – to provide a wide range of services to help people with diabetes. We rely mainly on voluntary donations to fund our research, campaigns and to provide information and support to help people living with diabetes.

If you would like to get involved and help bring about a better future for people with diabetes, please contact our Customer Services team on **020 7462 2791** and they will give you information about:

- Becoming a member of Diabetes UK
- Giving regular support to research through Diabetes UK Research Focus
- Making a donation
- Holding a fundraising event
- Giving through your payroll
- Including Diabetes UK in your will.

If you would like to become involved in any of Diabetes UK's fundraising activities, please get in touch with the Fundraising Department. You may wish to fundraise on your own or with friends, or to be associated with one of Diabetes UK's voluntary groups. The Fundraising Department can point you in whichever direction you prefer.

Your helpful advice and support and your own experiences of living with diabetes are essential to Diabetes UK's work, so do get in touch.

Research focus

Help us invest in diabetes research – join Diabetes UK Research Focus

Research Focus is Diabetes UK's regular giving scheme dedicated to funding diabetes research. Members of Research Focus each give a regular (monthly, quarterly or annual) amount. This means we can commit funds to long-term projects, knowing we will have the money to see the project through to its conclusion – a conclusion we hope will deliver real benefits for people with diabetes.

Members of Research Focus help fund research into the:

- Causes of diabetes
- Genetics of diabetes
- Secretion and action of insulin
- Control of diabetes
- Prevention and treatment of diabetes complications
- Treatment and care of people with diabetes
- Psychology of caring for diabetes.

Members of Research Focus give on a regular basis and so provide us with an ongoing source of funds to invest in diabetes research. Research Focus members who give £5 a month or more receive the annual Research Focus newsletter, an annual review, news items as and when diabetes research developments happen, and invitations to our Research Focus Forums where researchers discuss the projects they are working on.

People join Research Focus for a variety of reasons. Some recognise that though a cure for diabetes may be a long way off, it will never be reached if we don't invest in diabetes research now. Others value the potential benefits research may bring to the standard of diabetes care. Many parents with diabetes worry about the genetic link and hope for a day when we can accurately predict if their children will develop diabetes, so we can target future preventative treatments. Whatever the reason, Research Focus members all share the same belief – that research is the key to a better future for people with diabetes. One day, research may even lead us to a cure.

If you share this belief and would like to help achieve it, please contact us for further information about joining Diabetes UK Research Focus.

By letter: Research Focus Manager, Diabetes UK,
             10 Queen Anne St, London W1G 9LH

By phone: 020 7462 2791 (Customer Service Team)
By email: customerservice@diabetes.org.uk

■ How to join Diabetes UK

Diabetes UK is the charity for people with diabetes, working to improve their lives and to achieve our ultimate aim of a future without diabetes – something we could not do or hope for without our members.

Our members help us fund work to:

- ■ Provide **support and information** to people with diabetes so they are informed about their condition and are able to lead a full life.
- ■ **Campaign** for the rights and interests of people with diabetes to ensure they are not discriminated against because of their condition.
- ■ **Research** answers to the many questions that still surround diabetes and its complications, making progress towards our ultimate aim of a future without diabetes.

To become a member of Diabetes UK, please contact us for further information.

By letter: Diabetes UK, Customer Services,
            10 Queen Anne St, London W1G 9LH

By phone: 020 7462 2791
By email: customerservice@diabetes.org.uk

What membership of Diabetes UK gives you:

- Access to the latest, up-to-date information about diabetes care, research and other issues via our bi-monthly magazine *Balance*, and a wide range of information publications which we produce
- The opportunity to share their experiences with other people with diabetes through our support groups (over 400 nationwide)
- The ability to talk in confidence to Diabetes UK Careline about any diabetes issue or aspect of their diabetes (**020 7636 6112** during office hours)
- A range of insurance and financial products designed specifically with the needs of people with diabetes in mind.

■ National and regional offices

Diabetes UK aims to be closer to its members and to meet their needs as professionally as possible. To this end it has opened regional offices. By having an office in your area it can help ensure the best level of care for people with diabetes and that your voice is heard. Many of Diabetes UK's activities, such as research projects, holidays and network days, are local to your area.

Contact addresses

Diabetes UK
10 Queen Anne Street
London
W1G 9LH

Tel: 020 7323 1531
Fax: 020 7637 3644
Email: info@diabetes.org.uk

Diabetes UK Scotland
Savoy House
140 Sauchiehall Street
Glasgow
G2 3HD

Tel: 0141 332 2700
Fax: 0141 332 4880
Email: scotland@diabetes.org.uk

Diabetes UK North West
65 Bewsey Street
Warrington
WA2 7JQ

Tel: 01925 653 281
Fax: 01925 653 288
Email: n.west@diabetes.org.uk

Diabetes UK West Midlands
1 Eldon Court
Eldon Street
Walsall
WS1 2JP

Tel: 01922 614 500
Fax: 01922 646 789
Email: w.midlands@diabetes.org.uk

Diabetes UK Northern Ireland
John Gibson House
257 Lisburn Road
Belfast
BT9 7EN

Tel: 028 9066 6646
Fax: 028 9066 6333
Email: n.ireland@diabetes.org.uk

Diabetes UK Cymru
Quebec House
Castlebridge
Lowbridge Road East
Cardiff
CF11 9AB

Tel:01222 668 276
Fax: 01222 668 329
Email: wales@diabetes.org.uk

Diabetes UK Services

Diabetes UK Services is proud to offer a wide range of highly competitive insurance products that have been developed, in partnership with leading insurance broker Heath Lambert, specifically for people living with diabetes.

As a broker, Heath Lambert can negotiate directly with a range of insurers specifically on issues surrounding diabetes, meaning great deals on travel, motor and home insurance, and financial services.

For the first time, many people who would have previously been excluded will have access to some form of Critical Illness cover on a stand-alone basis.

All services can be reached through the one phone number with a dedicated team of professionals on the other end who understand the issues associated with diabetes.

blood tests *continued*
body mass index (BMI)   41–2
bread   2, 10, 22, 25, 28
bulk sweeteners   35
butter   26

Cakes   23, 26, 33
calcium   32
calluses   73, 75
calories   26, 35, 36
    high calorie foods   33, 37, 40
carbohydrate   2, 9, 23–5, 28, 34,
    37
    metabolism   10
    sources of   24–5, 30
cataracts   77, 78
causes
    of diabetes   2, 5–6, 15
cereals   10, 22, 25, 27
check-ups   18, 55
cheese   23, 26
chiropody   73, 82, 84
cholesterol   26–7, 71, 84
clinics, diabetic   52, 55, 80
coma *see* diabetic coma   6, 8, 17, 60
complications of diabetes   18,
    58–60
    affecting arteries   18, 70
    affecting eyes   17, 18, 77
    affecting feet   18, 71–6
    affecting kidneys   69, 79
    affecting nerves   69, 76, 77
    prevention of   2, 8, 21–2, 69
    and Social Security benefits   91
constipation   28
contact lenses   79
contraception   98–9
contraceptive pill   5, 98
control *see* diabetic control
cooking oils   26, 33
corns   73, 75
cortisone   59
cyclamates   36

dairy products   22, 23, 26, 32
dehydration   6
dentistry   80
diabetes (general references only)
    causes   2, 5–6, 15
    history   3
    how it develops   2–3
    numbers of cases   1, 3
    symptoms   5–6
    temporary   5
    types   4–5
    what it is   2
    see also Type 1 (insulin dependent)
    diabetes; Type 2 (non insulin
    dependent) diabetes
diabetes clinics   52, 55, 82
diabetic coma   6, 8, 17, 60
diabetes control
    checking it is effective   51–60
    during exercise   54, 93–4
    effect of illness   15, 79–80
    effect of soluble fibre   27, 30
    in hospital   80, 81–2
    loss of   58–9
    role of diabetic clinics   82
    when on insulin treatment
        64–6
Diabetes UK   1, 35, 40, 63, 68,
    89, 90, 93, 94, 97, 100,
    103–19
    campaigns   111
    care developments   105
    care inteventions   105–6
    Careline   104–5
    driving licence advice   68, 93
    employment advice   89, 110
    fundraising   112–13
    history   104
    insurance advice   89–90,
        110–11, 118–19
    Internet   108
    leaflets and magazines   107
    local groups   106, 111–12

membership 115–16
networks for healthcare
  professionals 108–9, 112
poster campaigns 109
regional offices 116–18
research 112–15
Social Security advice 91
St Vincent Declaration 112
travel guides 97
voluntary work for 94, 106,
  113–14
website 108
diabetic foods 36, 42
diabetic retinopathy 18, 77
Diabur-Test 5000 56
diarrhoea 60, 77
Diastix 56
diet 7, 9–10, 21–43
  adjusting 22
  basic guidelines 23, 29
  eating out 38–9, 97
  foods to be eaten freely 23
  foods to be restricted 23
  on holiday 97
  with insulin treatment 7, 66
  with tablet treatment 4, 7,
    48, 49
  for the whole family 22, 42–3
  see also foods; meals; snacks
dieting to lose weight 22, 27, 40–3
  effect on blood cholesterol 26
  effect of exercise 22, 93–4
  restricting alcohol intake 39–40
  restricting high calorie food
    27, 37
  role of high fibre foods 27–8
  target weight 22, 42, 58
digestion and metabolism 10
discrimination, fighting 109–11
diuretics (water tablets) 5, 59, 80
drinks 10, 16, 25, 33, 36
  see also alcohol

driving
  effect of low alcohol drinks 40
  HGV licences 68, 92–3, 110
  and hypoglycaemia 50,
    66–7, 68
  informing DVLA 67, 91
  licence applications 91–3
  motor insurance 67, 89, 91
  passenger-carrying vehicle
    licences 68, 92–3
  when on insulin treatment
    66–7
  when on tablet treatment
    50, 93
drugs
  affecting diabetic control 59, 80
  revealing pre-existing diabetes 5

eating out 38–9, 95
eggs 23, 31
employers, attitudes to diabetes
  88–9
employment *see* work
energy
  breakdown of body energy
    quantity in foods 38
  stores 13, 16, 17, 37
  sources of 2, 10, 11, 37
ethnic origin 4, 15–16
exercise
  effect on blood glucose 2, 13,
    54, 93
  effect on blood pressure 71
  importance 22, 43, 93–4
  quantity 43
  types of 44–5
  when on insulin treatment 66
  when on tablet treatment 93
eyes 69, 77–9
eye tests 17, 78, 91
  see also vision

family
    chances of them developing
        diabetes 5–6, 15, 99
    their feelings about your
        diabetes 99–100
fat 9, 13, 23, 31
    effect of soluble fibre 27
    metabolism 10, 16
    quantity in food 38
    reducing intake of 22, 37,
        42–3
    sources 26, 32–3
    types 26–7
feelings, about your diabetes
    99–100
feet
    examining and inspecting 73
    first aid for 75
    foot problems 18, 21, 69
    nail cutting 73
    protecting from heat and cold 74
    rules for foot care 72–4
        for older people 73
    washing 74
fibre, dietary 27–8, 30, 31
fish 26
flour 28
fluid, excessive loss of 17, 60
food
    basic components 23–9
    diabetic 36, 42
    digestion and metabolism 10
    high calorie 27, 37
    high fibre 22, 27–8
    starchy 2, 22, 24, 25, 28, 30
    sugary 22, 24, 25, 29, 32–4, 66
    see also carbohydrate; fat; protein;
    diet; meals; snacks
food labels 35–6
fructosamine test 54, 83
fructose 35
fruit 22, 23, 27, 30–1, 35
fruit juice 31, 49

gastroenteritis 59, 96
genitals, itching and sore 6, 16
gestational diabetes 16
glitazones 47, 48, 50
glucose see blood glucose
Glycaemic Index (GI) 34–5
glycosuria 14

habits, altering 8, 23
Haemoglobin A_{1c} test 54, 83
heart disease 21, 38
heredity 4, 6, 15, 99
HGV licences 68, 92–3, 110
high calorie foods 27, 37
high fibre foods 22, 27–8
holidays 95–7
    holidays for young people 105
    foreign food 97
    insurance 90, 110
hospital admission 60, 81–2
hyperglycaemia (high blood
        glucose) 2, 14, 15
    long-term effects of 2, 18, 48, 69
    symptoms 16–17
hypertension see blood pressure,
    high
hypo see hypoglycaemia
hypoglycaemia (low blood
        glucose) 48–9, 65, 66–7
    and driving 50, 66–7
    insulin reaction 65
    treatment 49

identity card 96
illness
    associated illnesses 80
    and discovery of diabetes 3, 5, 17
    effect on blood sugar levels
        2, 5, 15, 59
    effect on diabetic control
        15, 65, 79–80

illness *continued*
   sickness insurance   90
   urine testing during   54
   when travelling or on holiday   96
impotence   76
incontinence   16
infection   16, 59
injections *see* insulin treatment
injuries and accidents   5, 13, 15
   insurance   90
insoluble fibre   27, 28
insulin
   discovery   3
   driving licence application and
     91–3
   function   2
   how it works   2, 12–13, 64–5
   injections *see* insulin treatment
   not working effectively   2, 12–15
   too little being produced   15
insulin dependent diabetes *see* Type 1
   (insulin dependent) diabetes
insulin treatment
   in Type 1 (insulin dependent)
   diabetes   7, 63
   in Type 2 (non insulin dependent)
   diabetes   4, 7, 22, 63–8
     dosage   66
     duration   65–6
     temporary   65, 81
     too much   65
insulin-producing cells   3, 4, 12
insulin reaction *see* hypoglycaemia
insurance   18, 89–90
   discrimination   110–11
   holiday   90, 96
   life   90, 110
   motor   67, 89, 91, 111
   travel   110
islets of Langerhans   3, 12
itching, of the genitals   6, 16

Jobs *see* work
juvenile diabetes *see* Type 1
   (insulin dependent) diabetes

Ketoacidosis *see* diabetic coma
kidney damage   21, 69, 79
kilocalories *see* calories

Lens of the eye   17, 18, 77
life assurance   90, 110
liver   2, 10, 80
long-term effects of diabetes   18, 48
   on arteries   21, 70
   on eyes   77–8
   on feet   69
   on kidneys   69, 79
   on nerves   69, 77
   prevention of   2, 21–2, 69
   and Social Security benefits   91

Maturity onset diabetes *see* Type 2
   (non insulin dependent) diabetes
meals
   eating regularly   22, 42, 66
   effect on blood sugar levels
     2, 3, 9, 12, 64
   foreign food   97
   see also diet; food; snacks
meat   23, 26, 31
medical check-ups   18, 55
medical review   82–4
medication *see* drugs; tablet
   treatment
metabolism   10–11
meters, blood glucose   57
metformin   47, 48, 49
milk   23, 26, 32
minerals   28
monounsaturated fats   26, 27, 33

motor insurance 67, 89, 91, 111
mouth, dry 6, 16
mumps as cause of diabetes 5

nail cutting 71
needles 64
nephropathy *see* kidney damage
neuritis *see* neuropathy
neuropathy 71–2, 73, 76
non insulin dependent diabetes
    see Type 2 (non insulin dependent)
    diabetes
normoglycaemia 14
Nutrasweet™ 36
nutritive sweeteners 35

Overweight
    causes 15, 22
    effect on blood cholesterol 26
    effect on insulin activity 13,
        15, 22, 66
    increased chances of developing
    Type 2 (non insulin dependent)
        diabetes 4, 5, 6, 15
    weight chart 41
        see also dieting to lose weight

Pancreas 3, 12
    diseases of 5, 80
    not producing enough insulin
        13, 15, 16
    reaction to changes in blood
sugar levels 12, 22
pancreatitis 5
passenger-carrying vehicle
    licences 68, 92–3
pasta 10, 22, 25, 28
pastry 23, 26
pensions 90
polyols 35

polyunsaturated fats 26, 27
potatoes 2, 10, 22, 25
prandial glucose regulators
    47, 50
prednisolone 59
pregnancy, diabetes in 16, 66,
    98–9
prescription charges 90
prevention
    of arterial disease 21, 70
    of complications 2, 8, 21–2, 69
    of eye damage 78
    of foot problems 72–3
    of hypoglycaemia 65
protein 9
    metabolism 10, 16
    sources 25, 31
pulses 22, 25, 31

Quorn 31

records
    blood tests 58
    urine tests 55
renal threshold 14–15, 52–3
retina 18, 77–8
retinopathy, diabetic 18, 77
retirement 84–5
rice 10, 22, 25, 28
roughage *see* fibre

Saccharin 34
salt 23, 36, 60
saturated fats 26, 27, 33
shoes 72, 75
sickness insurance 90
smoking 71, 72, 85
snacks 26, 30, 31, 66
    during exercise 93

effect on blood glucose levels 3, 12, 65
see also diet; food; meals
Social Security 91
sodium 37, 38
soluble fibre 27, 30, 31
soya products 31
sport *see* exercise
St Vincent Declaration 112
starchy foods 2, 22, 24, 25, 28, 30
steroid drugs 5, 59, 80
stress 13, 15, 54, 59
sugar
 alternatives to 33–4
 controlling intake of 22, 23, 25, 33, 66
 Glycaemic Index (GI) 34–5
 quantities in foods 37, 38
 see also blood glucose
sulphonylureas 47, 48, 49
superannuation 90
swallowing, difficulty in 16
sweeteners, artificial 36
 intense 36
 non-intense 35
symptoms 5–6, 16–17
 elimination of 2, 21
 of hyperglycaemia 16–17
 of hypoglycaemia 46–7, 65
 lack of 7, 18, 22, 51
syringes 64

tablet treatment 47–50
 alcohol and 40
 with diet treatment 4, 7, 48
 names of tablets 47
 not working effectively 48, 59
 side-effects 48–50
 when to take tablets 22, 48
target weight 22, 42, 58

test strips 57
thirst 6, 16, 51, 79
thrush 16
tiredness 6, 17
toenail cutting 73
tofu 31
travel 95–7
 foreign food 97
 illness 96
 insurance 96, 110
treatment
 abandoning treatment 59
 alternative treatment 50
 checking it is effective 8, 51–60
 diet treatment *see* diet
 for eye damage 78
 for hypoglycaemia 49
 of illnesses other than diabetes 80
 importance of 8, 18, 21, 51, 64
 insulin *see* insulin treatment
 tablet *see* tablet treatment
 types 7–8
 what it is designed to do 2, 8, 17, 21, 64
Type 1 (insulin dependent) diabetes 4
 cause 4
 heredity 5, 99
 symptoms 6–7
 treatment 7
 who gets it 5
Type 2 (non insulin dependent) diabetes 4
 diet treatment 4, 21–45
 effect on blood glucose levels *see* hypoglycaemia
 heredity 4, 5, 15, 99
 insulin treatment 4, 7, 22, 63–4
 long-term effects 18, 69–79
 loss of control 58–60

symptomless   7, 18, 51
symptoms   6, 16–17
tablet treatment   47–50
what causes it   4, 15
who gets it   4, 15–16
world distribution   15

Urine
   blood glucose in   14–15, 16, 51
   difficulty in passing   77
   passing large amounts of
      6, 16, 51, 79
urine tests   15, 65
   compared with blood tests
      51–2, 65
   frequency   54
   high   52, 54
   on holiday   96
   for kidney damage   79
   how they work   52, 53
   how to do them   56
   negative   52, 54
   positive   54
   records   55–6
   test strips   57
   when to do them   55

Vaccinations   80, 97
vegetables   22, 23, 27, 30–1, 39
Viagra   76
vision see also eyes
   blurring   6, 17, 78, 84
   deteriorating   77
vitamins   28
vomiting   6, 17, 59, 60

Water tablets see diuretics
weakness   17
weighing, regular   58
weight chart   41
weight loss
   deliberate see dieting to
      lose weight
   symptom of diabetes
      6, 17, 40, 51, 59
work   8, 87–9
   jobs imposing restrictions
      68, 87–8
   when on insulin treatment
      66, 67–8

Yoghurt   29

Index compiled by Annette Musker